ɔrary
ʻedical Associa

Fifty Neurologic Cases
From Mayo Clinic

Fifty Neurologic Cases
From Mayo Clinic

Edited by

John H. Noseworthy, MD, FRCPC

Chair, Department of Neurology, Mayo Clinic;
Professor of Neurology, Mayo Clinic College of Medicine;
Rochester, Minnesota, USA

OXFORD
UNIVERSITY PRESS

2004

OXFORD
UNIVERSITY PRESS

Oxford   New York
Auckland   Bangkok   Buenos Aires   Cape Town   Chennai
Dar es Salaam   Delhi   Hong Kong   Istanbul   Karachi   Kolkata
Kuala Lumpur   Madrid   Melbourne   Mexico City   Mumbai   Nairobi
São Paulo   Shanghai   Taipei   Tokyo   Toronto

The triple-shield Mayo logo and the words MAYO and MAYO CLINIC are marks of Mayo
Foundation for Medical Education and Research.

Copyright © 2004 by Mayo Foundation for Medical Education and Research

Published by Oxford University Press, Inc.
198 Madison Avenue, New York, New York 10016
www.oup.com

Oxford is a registered trademark of Oxford University Press

This book was designed and typeset by Mayo Foundation for Medical Education and Research.

Care has been taken to confirm the accuracy of the information presented and to describe generally accepted practices. However, the authors, editor, and publisher are not responsible for errors
or omissions or for any consequences from application of the information in this book and make
no warranty, expressed or implied, with respect to the contents of the publication. This book
should not be used apart from the advice of a qualified health care provider.

The authors, editor, and publisher have exerted efforts to ensure that drug selection and dosage
set forth in this text are in accordance with current recommendations and practice at the time of
publication. However, in view of ongoing research, changes in government regulations, and the
constant flow of information relating to drug therapy and drug reactions, the reader is urged to
check the package insert for each drug for any change in indications and dosage and for added
warnings and precautions. This is particularly important when the recommended agent is a
new or infrequently used drug.

Some drugs and medical devices presented in this publication have U.S. Food and Drug
Administration (FDA) clearance for limited use in restricted research settings. It is the respon-
sibility of health care providers to ascertain the FDA status of each drug or device planned for
use in their clinical practice.

Library of Congress Cataloging-in-Publication Data
Fifty neurologic cases from Mayo Clinic / edited by John H. Noseworthy.
p. ; cm. Includes index.
ISBN 0-19-517744-4 (cloth) —ISBN 0-19-517745-2 (pbk)
1. Neurology—Case studies.
[DNLM: 1. Nervous System Diseases—diagnosis—United States—Case Reports. 2. Nervous
System Diseases—diagnosis—United States—Problems and Exercises. 3. Neurology—meth-
ods—United States—Case Reports. 4. Neurology—methods—United States—Problems and
Exercises. WL 141 F469 2004] I. Noseworthy, John H. II. Mayo Clinic.
RC359.F545 2004 616.8'0475--dc22 2004043453

9 8 7 6 5 4 3 2 1

Printed in the United States of America
on acid-free paper

Credits

The cases described herein have been published previously:

Case 12—Klein CJ, Boes CJ, Chapin JE, *et al*. Adult polyglucosan body disease: case description of an expanding genetic and clinical syndrome. *Muscle Nerve* 2004;**29**:323-8. By permission of Wiley Periodicals.

Case 22—Capobianco DJ. Facial pain as a symptom of nonmetastatic lung cancer. *Headache* 1995;**35**:581-5. By permission of the American Headache Society.

Case 30—Petty GW, Engel AG, Younge BR, *et al*. Retinocochleocerebral vasculopathy. *Medicine (Baltimore)* 1998;**77**:12-40. By permission of Williams & Wilkins.

Case 33—Kumar N, Gross JB Jr, Ahlskog JE. Myelopathy due to copper deficiency. *Neurology* 2003;**61**:273-4. By permission of the American Academy of Neurology.

Case 40—Black DF, Swanson JW. A case of familial hemiplegic migraine and Erdheim-Chester disease (abstract). *Headache* 2002;**42**:460-1. By permission of the American Headache Society; Black DF, Kung S, Sola CL, *et al*. Familial hemiplegic migraine, neuropsychiatric symptoms, and Erdheim-Chester disease. *Headache* (in press). By permission of the American Headache Society.

Case 44—Bekavac I, Halloran JI. Meningocele-induced positional syncope and retinal hemorrhage. *AJNR Am J Neuroradiol* 2003;**24**:838-9. By permission of the American Society of Neuroradiology.

The cover illustration shows the carillon tower on top the Plummer Building of Mayo Clinic in Rochester, Minnesota. When this building was completed in 1928, it was the tallest building in Minnesota, at a height of 297 feet. This Romanesque building has many wonderful architectural features, including massive solid bronze entrance doors of Moorish design. Each door weighs 4,000 lb and is elaborately decorated with square panels that symbolize life in Minnesota, including education, domestic arts, mechanical and fine arts and sciences, agriculture, and Native American culture. Representative icons and other architectural features of the Plummer Building punctuate the end of the cases.

Dedication

To my friends in the Department of Neurology at Mayo Clinic, who, by their example, teach me daily how to better meet the needs of my patients.

Preface and Acknowledgments

The desire to publish *Fifty Neurologic Cases From Mayo Clinic* arose from the splendid example provided by Doctors Adrian J. Wills and C. David Marsden in their book, *Fifty Neurological Cases from the National Hospital.* Their collection of informative cases from Queen Square is a fitting tribute to a timeless institution. At Mayo Clinic, we, too, are proud of our rich tradition of neurologic excellence spanning nearly a century, beginning in 1913 when Doctor Walter D. "Pops" Sheldon joined the staff. He was soon joined by Doctors Henry W. Woltman and Frederick P. Moersch and, thereafter, by many other distinguished neurologists.

Neurologists enjoy evaluating patients who have difficult diagnostic problems. In the years since moving from the University of Western Ontario in London, Canada, to Mayo Clinic, I have been challenged daily by complex cases from near and far. I have been privileged to experience the camaraderie of wonderful colleagues in neurology and neurosurgery. Their tireless commitment to their patients and their example are beyond comparison. I am grateful to them for contributing their cases and their scholarly commentaries to this little book.

I would also like to thank the fine editorial staff of the Section of Scientific Publications of Mayo Clinic and my able secretary Melissa L. Fenske for their assistance.

I hope that the readers will be challenged by these cases and learn from the master clinicians in our department at Mayo.

John H. Noseworthy, MD, FRCPC
Rochester, Minnesota, December 2003

Contents

List of Contributors

Charles H. Adler, MD
Chair, Division of Movement Disorders and Consultant, Department of Neurology, Mayo Clinic, Scottsdale, Arizona; Professor of Neurology, Mayo Clinic College of Medicine, Rochester, Minnesota

Allen J. Aksamit, MD
Consultant, Department of Neurology, Mayo Clinic; Associate Professor of Neurology, Mayo Clinic College of Medicine; Rochester, Minnesota

Raymond G. Auger, MD
Consultant, Department of Neurology, Mayo Clinic; Associate Professor of Neurology, Mayo Clinic College of Medicine; Rochester, Minnesota

David F. Black, MD
Senior Associate Consultant, Department of Neurology, Mayo Clinic; Instructor in Neurology, Mayo Clinic College of Medicine; Rochester, Minnesota

Christopher J. Boes, MD
Consultant, Division of Regional Neurology, Mayo Clinic; Assistant Professor of Neurology, Mayo Clinic College of Medicine; Rochester, Minnesota

Bradley F. Boeve, MD
Chair, Division of Behavioral Neurology, Mayo Clinic; Associate Professor of Neurology, Mayo Clinic College of Medicine; Rochester, Minnesota

E. Peter Bosch, MD
Consultant, Department of Neurology, Mayo Clinic, Scottsdale, Arizona; Professor of Neurology, Mayo Clinic College of Medicine; Rochester, Minnesota

James H. Bower, MD
Consultant, Division of Regional Neurology, Mayo Clinic; Assistant Professor of Neurology, Mayo Clinic College of Medicine, Rochester, Minnesota

Paul W. Brazis, MD
Consultant, Department of Ophthalmology, Mayo Clinic, Jacksonville, Florida; Professor of Neurology, Mayo Clinic College of Medicine, Rochester, Minnesota

Robert D. Brown, Jr., MD
Chair, Division of Cerebrovascular Diseases, Mayo Clinic; Associate Professor of Neurology, Mayo Clinic College of Medicine; Rochester, Minnesota

David J. Capobianco, MD
Consultant, Department of Neurology, Mayo Clinic, Jacksonville, Florida; Assistant Professor of Neurology, Mayo Clinic College of Medicine, Rochester, Minnesota

Gregory D. Cascino, MD
Chair, Division of Epilepsy, Mayo Clinic; Professor of Neurology, Mayo Clinic College of Medicine; Rochester, Minnesota

Richard J. Caselli, MD
Chair, Department of Neurology, Mayo Clinic, Scottsdale, Arizona; Professor of Neurology, Mayo Clinic College of Medicine, Rochester, Minnesota

William P. Cheshire, MD
Consultant, Department of Neurology, Mayo Clinic, Jacksonville, Florida; Associate Professor of Neurology, Mayo Clinic College of Medicine, Rochester, Minnesota

Shelley A. Cross, MD
Consultant, Department of Neurology, Mayo Clinic; Assistant Professor of Neurology, Mayo Clinic College of Medicine; Rochester, Minnesota

Brian A. Crum, MD
Consultant, Division of Clinical Neurophysiology, Mayo Clinic; Assistant Professor of Neurology, Mayo Clinic College of Medicine; Rochester, Minnesota

Jasper R. Daube, MD
Consultant, Department of Neurology, Mayo Clinic; Professor of Neurology, Mayo Clinic College of Medicine; Rochester, Minnesota

David W. Dodick, MD
Consultant, Department of Neurology, Mayo Clinic, Scottsdale, Arizona; Associate Professor of Neurology, Mayo Clinic College of Medicine, Rochester, Minnesota

Joseph F. Drazkowski, MD
Senior Associate Consultant, Department of Neurology, Mayo Clinic, Scottsdale, Arizona; Assistant Professor of Neurology, Mayo Clinic College of Medicine, Rochester, Minnesota

P. James B. Dyck, MD
Consultant, Department of Neurology, Mayo Clinic; Assistant Professor of Neurology, Mayo Clinic College of Medicine; Rochester, Minnesota

Peter J. Dyck, MD
Consultant, Department of Neurology, Mayo Clinic; Roy E. and Merle Meyer Professor of Neuroscience and Professor of Neurology, Mayo Clinic College of Medicine; Rochester, Minnesota

Andrew G. Engel, MD
Consultant, Department of Neurology, Mayo Clinic; William L. McKnight–3M Professor of Neuroscience and Professor of Neurology, Mayo Clinic College of Medicine; Rochester, Minnesota

Kelly D. Flemming, MD
Consultant, Department of Neurology, Mayo Clinic; Assistant Professor of Neurology, Mayo Clinic College of Medicine; Rochester, Minnesota

C. Michel Harper, Jr., MD
Consultant, Department of Neurology, Mayo Clinic; Professor of Neurology, Mayo Clinic College of Medicine; Rochester, Minnesota

Keith A. Josephs, MD
Senior Associate Consultant, Department of Neurology, Mayo Clinic; Assistant Professor of Neurology, Mayo Clinic College of Medicine; Rochester Minnesota

David W. Kimmel, MD
Consultant, Department of Neurology, Mayo Clinic; Associate Professor of Neurology, Mayo Clinic College of Medicine; Rochester, Minnesota

Christopher J. Klein, MD
Senior Associate Consultant, Department of Neurology, Mayo Clinic; Assistant Professor of Neurology, Mayo Clinic College of Medicine; Rochester, Minnesota

William E. Krauss, MD
Consultant, Department of Neurologic Surgery, Mayo Clinic; Assistant Professor of Neurosurgery, Mayo Clinic College of Medicine; Rochester, Minnesota

Neeraj Kumar, MD
Senior Associate Consultant, Department of Neurology, Mayo Clinic; Assistant Professor of Neurology, Mayo Clinic College of Medicine; Rochester, Minnesota

Nancy L. Kuntz, MD
Consultant, Division of Child and Adolescent Neurology, Mayo Clinic; Assistant Professor of Neurology, Mayo Clinic College of Medicine; Rochester, Minnesota

Claudia F. Lucchinetti, MD
Consultant, Department of Neurology, Mayo Clinic; Associate Professor of Neurology, Mayo Clinic College of Medicine; Rochester, Minnesota

Kenneth J. Mack, MD

Senior Associate Consultant, Department of Neurology, Mayo Clinic; Associate Professor of Neurology, Mayo Clinic College of Medicine; Rochester, Minnesota

Irene Meissner, MD

Consultant, Department of Neurology, Mayo Clinic; Associate Professor of Neurology, Mayo Clinic College of Medicine; Rochester, Minnesota

Bahram Mokri, MD

Consultant, Department of Neurology, Mayo Clinic; Professor of Neurology, Mayo Clinic College of Medicine; Rochester, Minnesota

Manfred D. Muenter, MD

Emeritus Member, Department of Neurology, Mayo Clinic, Scottsdale, Arizona; Emeritus Professor of Neurology, Mayo Clinic College of Medicine, Rochester, Minnesota

John H. Noseworthy, MD

Chair, Department of Neurology, Mayo Clinic; Professor of Neurology, Mayo Clinic College of Medicine; Rochester, Minnesota

Ronald C. Petersen, MD

Consultant, Department of Neurology, Mayo Clinic; Cora Kanow Professor of Alzheimer's Disease Research and Professor of Neurology, Mayo Clinic College of Medicine; Rochester, Minnesota

George W. Petty, MD

Consultant, Department of Neurology, Mayo Clinic; Associate Professor of Neurology, Mayo Clinic College of Medicine; Rochester, Minnesota

Deborah L. Renaud, MD

Senior Associate Consultant, Department of Neurology, Mayo Clinic; Instructor in Neurology, Mayo Clinic College of Medicine; Rochester, Minnesota

Moses Rodriguez, MD

Chair, Section of Multiple Sclerosis and Consultant, Department of Immunology, Mayo Clinic; Mildred A. and Henry Uihlein II Professor of Medical Research and Professor of Neurology and Immunology, Mayo Clinic College of Medicine; Rochester, Minnesota

Frank A. Rubino, MD

Consultant, Department of Neurology, Mayo Clinic, Jacksonville, Florida; Professor of Neurology, Mayo Clinic College of Medicine, Rochester, Minnesota

Paola Sandroni, MD
   Consultant, Department of Neurology, Mayo Clinic; Assistant
   Professor of Neurology, Mayo Clinic College of Medicine;
   Rochester, Minnesota
Duygu Selcen, MD
   Senior Associate Consultant, Department of Neurology, Mayo Clinic;
   Assistant Professor of Neurology, Mayo Clinic College of Medicine;
   Rochester, Minnesota
Michael H. Silber, MB, ChB
   Consultant, Department of Neurology and Sleep Disorders Center,
   Mayo Clinic; Associate Professor of Neurology, Mayo Clinic College
   of Medicine; Rochester, Minnesota
Michael Sinnreich, MD
   Peripheral Nerve Fellow, Mayo Graduate School of Medicine,
   Rochester, Minnesota
Joseph I. Sirven, MD
   Consultant, Department of Neurology, Mayo Clinic, Scottsdale,
   Arizona; Associate Professor of Neurology, Mayo Clinic College of
   Medicine, Rochester, Minnesota
Guillermo A. Suarez, MD
   Consultant, Department of Neurology, Mayo Clinic; Assistant
   Professor of Neurology, Mayo Clinic College of Medicine;
   Rochester, Minnesota
Jerry W. Swanson, MD
   Chair, Division of Headache, Mayo Clinic; Professor of Neurology,
   Mayo Clinic College of Medicine; Rochester, Minnesota
Joon H. Uhm, MD
   Consultant, Department of Neurology, Mayo Clinic; Assistant
   Professor of Neurology, Mayo Clinic College of Medicine;
   Rochester, Minnesota
Ryan J. Uitti, MD
   Consultant, Department of Neurology, Mayo Clinic, Jacksonville,
   Florida; Professor of Neurology, Mayo Clinic College of Medicine,
   Rochester, Minnesota
Steven Vernino, MD
   Consultant, Department of Neurology, Mayo Clinic; Assistant
   Professor of Neurology, Mayo Clinic College of Medicine;
   Rochester, Minnesota
Eelco F. M. Wijdicks, MD
   Chair, Division of Critical Care Neurology, Mayo Clinic; Professor of
   Neurology, Mayo Clinic College of Medicine; Rochester, Minnesota

Introduction

This book is designed both to teach and to entertain. The format is simple. Fifty informative cases are presented succinctly with an emphasis on the critical aspects of each case (history, examination, investigations). The authors were given the challenge of including not more than one or two figures or tables and one reference. Just enough information has been presented in the title of each case (see the Table of Contents) and in the text to permit the reader to localize the lesion, identify the likely family of disorders (e.g., vascular, infectious, metabolic, degenerative, neoplastic), and, depending on the neurologic sophistication of the reader, to reach the correct diagnosis. When ready, the reader turns the page and is treated to a brief Commentary by a Mayo Clinic neurologist addressing the important elements of the case and the specific disease process. As such, the puzzle is presented and the solution revealed.

These cases present a graded challenge to our colleagues in medicine. Students and residents should find the exercise in localization and differential diagnosis to be both fun and stimulating. Physicians with considerable neurologic expertise (internists, psychiatrists, rehabilitation physicians, pediatricians, and geriatricians) will particularly appreciate the commentaries. Finally, neurologists and neurosurgeons will enjoy the full challenge of matching wits directly with the discussants. In doing so, perhaps readers will recall similar cases that have challenged them in their practice.

This little book will enhance learning for readers at each stage of their careers. Young students soon learn that clinical medicine in general, and neurology in particular, requires precision in extracting an accurate history and correctly identifying the abnormal physical findings. Neurology probably demonstrates as well as any medical specialty the breadth and precision of the examination and the value of this technique in localizing the site of the lesion. The medical student learns the essential elements of these tasks and, with proper mentoring and much practice, gradually develops proficiency. The resident and fellow learn to clarify and quantify the pertinent positive and negative features that characterize each case. For generations, neurologists have taught wisely that the combination of the temporal profile of the illness (i.e., acute, subacute, or chronic) and the presence or absence of focal signs informs on the likely pathogenesis (e.g., neoplastic, vascular, or degenerative disorder). These key elements are demonstrated in every case in this book.

As we mature as physicians, we learn the art of presenting our cases to our colleagues in an abbreviated and clearly focused manner. This ability to crystallize all the elements of a complex case into a few informative sentences demonstrates our maturity and competence as clearly as anything we do as physicians. In neurology, this skill enables the analytical listener to determine whether the patient has a neurologic disorder and to localize the site(s) of the lesion, to deduce the probable pathophysiologic process, to formulate a differential diagnosis, and to make the diagnosis. With these steps, the neurologist determines the studies that are needed to confirm the correct diagnosis. The format that has been selected for the book illustrates the value of this exercise in a manner that reflects the daily practice of neurology.

The cases have been selected to span child and adult neurology to demonstrate the spectrum of problems seen in an office practice. Several cases have unique features (e.g., a child with recurrent aseptic meningitis, arthropathy, deafness, and rash; an adult with drenching sweats, sleep talking, and weight loss). Others share a superficial similarity to emphasize the diversity of cases that may have a similar signature (e.g., intermittent diplopia and progressive ataxia). Finally, the commentaries, although brief, discuss the important points of differential diagnosis and recent advances in the understanding of the disorders responsible for each patient's illness.

The hope is that readers will enjoy these cases and, in doing so, will find lessons that will assist them in the care of their patients.

JHN

Fifty Neurologic Cases
From Mayo Clinic

History

At age 52 years, a left-handed man began experiencing difficulties stating the names of familiar people and objects. Initially, he had no apparent problems with memory or other cognitive functions or changes in behavior. By age 54, difficulties with verbal comprehension had developed, but he still worked as a farmer and had no problem working or driving. At age 55, he developed a profound interest in listening to polka music, sometimes doing so for 12 hours or more at a time. By age 57, he was not able to read or write or to recognize most familiar faces and objects.

His father and paternal aunt had become forgetful late in life. His son has congenital apraxia of speech that has improved markedly with speech therapy.

Examination

Neurologic examination at age 53 revealed an alert, cooperative man whose language was fluent. He had difficulty naming simple objects and famous faces. Reading, writing, memory, and constructional praxis were all preserved. Over the next 4 years, his aphasia worsened, as did recognition of words, objects, and faces (associative agnosia). His verbal memory and attention also declined; yet, on examination at age 57, his recall of where objects were hidden in the office and his ability to draw figures remained intact.

Investigations

The cerebrospinal fluid examination was normal. Serial magnetic resonance imaging demonstrated progressive left, and then right, anterior temporal lobe atrophy (Figure). Initial neuropsychologic testing at age 53 demonstrated problems with divided attention, mental manipulation, executive functioning, and verbal learning and recall; his performance on language function tests (e.g., Boston Naming Test [BNT] score of 16/60) was particularly poor. Subsequent testing sessions showed progression in all cognitive domains, particularly language (BNT, 3/60 at age 56); yet, his copy of the Rey-Osterreith Complex Figure was almost perfect.

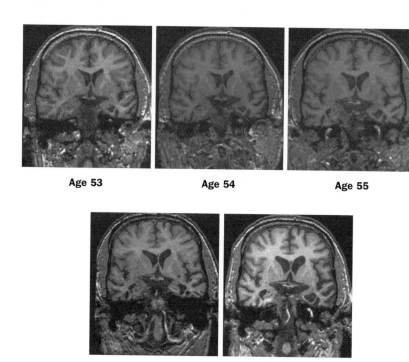

Age 53   **Age 54**   **Age 55**

Age 56   **Age 57**

FIGURE. Representative T_1-weighted coronal magnetic resonance images of patient from age 53 to 57 years. Note the progressive atrophy of the left amygdala and temporal cortex beginning at age 53. Atrophy in the right amygdala and temporal cortex was subtle at age 54, but it was clearly progressive over the years. (From Boeve BF, Geda YE. *Neurology* 2001;**57**:1485. By permission of the American Academy of Neurology.)

Commentary by Dr. Bradley F. Boeve

The terms "semantic dementia," "semantic aphasia and associative agnosia," "primary progressive aphasia," "chronic progressive aphasia," "temporal variant of frontotemporal dementia," and "focal or asymmetric cortical degeneration syndrome" have all been applied to patients who exhibit a degenerative neurobehavioral disorder with progressive impairment predominantly or exclusively in the domain of language. When impairment is isolated to language, the term "primary progressive aphasia" is appropriate; when impairment is present in object naming (i.e., anomia) *and* word meaning (i.e., agnosia), with other aspects of language and cognition relatively intact, the term "semantic dementia" is apt. The initial symptom is typically "forgetfulness for names," and although paraphasic errors, dyslexia, dysgraphia, visual agnosia, and executive dysfunction usually evolve with time, many patients perform daily activities remarkably well over the initial 2 to 5 years of symptoms. Progression can vary, with symptoms reflecting the topography of progressive cortical dysfunction. Typically, degeneration spreads posteriorly in the ipsilateral temporal lobe, with involvement eventually extending to the perisylvian, frontosubcortical, and sometimes superior parietal regions in the dominant hemisphere. When the contralateral hemisphere is affected, a remarkably consistent finding is progressive atrophy in the opposite anterior temporal lobe. If and when sufficient nondominant hemisphere frontotemporal cerebral dysfunction ensues, problematic neuropsychiatric features can evolve, such as socially inappropriate, disinhibited, and even criminal behavior. Misidentification errors, prosopagnosia, and ultimately multimodal associative agnosia become apparent as the nondominant temporal lobe atrophies.

Semantic dementia is one of the focal or asymmetric cortical degeneration syndromes and is associated with anterior temporal lobe dysfunction. Other clinical syndromes include progressive nonfluent aphasia associated with dominant hemisphere frontal opercular or insular dysfunction; frontotemporal dementia associated with dorsolateral prefrontal, orbitofrontal, or anterior cingulate dysfunction (or a combination of these); corticobasal syndrome associated with parieto-frontal cortical dysfunction; and posterior cortical atrophy associated with parieto-occipital cortical dysfunction. Although the nomenclature for these syndromes and the disorders that underlie them can be confusing, the conceptual perspective is the same—symptomatology is dictated more by the topography of dysfunction than by the underlying histopathologic disorder.

The pathologic substrates for semantic dementia have tended to be associated with either nonspecific neurodegenerative changes (e.g., "dementia lacking distinctive histopathology" or "frontotemporal lobar degeneration" with or without ubiquitin-positive inclusions) or a disorder within the tauopathy spectrum (e.g., Pick's disease, corticobasal degeneration, or argyrophilic brain disease). Alzheimer's disease rarely presents in this manner. Mutations in the *tau* gene have been identified in some patients who present with semantic dementia. No therapy has been identified that alters the pathophysiologic mechanism of the disorders that manifest as semantic dementia, nor have pharmacologic manipulations led to a marked and sustained symptomatic benefit in any patient. Speech therapy is reasonable for patients early in the course of the disease.

A striking and poorly understood observation is the remarkable evolution of artistic talent in rare persons with frontotemporal dementia, of whom some have had semantic dementia. Some patients have produced paintings more elaborate than their past renderings, whereas others have developed interests in listening to or playing forms of music that previously had not been considered interesting. This phenomenon seems completely contrary to degenerative brain disease. Whether compensatory mechanisms in relatively unaffected neuronal networks or disinhibition of affected neuronal networks (or both) explains this phenomenon is not known. Further study in semantic dementia and other focal or asymmetric cortical degeneration syndromes may not only improve our understanding of degenerative brain disease but also provide insight into the neurologic underpinnings of artistic appreciation and expression.

REFERENCE

Neary D, Snowden J, Gustafson L, *et al*. Frontotemporal lobar degeneration: a consensus on clinical diagnostic criteria. *Neurology* 1998;**51**:1546-54.

History

A 30-year-old man first developed trouble arising from the floor and climbing stairs during puberty. Through adolescence, he had a progressive decrease in academic and athletic performance. At age 20, he had a manic episode with paranoia. Over the next 10 years, he had multiple psychiatric hospitalizations for episodes of psychosis, mania, and depression that were relatively refractory to medication. Also, he developed progressive slurred speech, trouble swallowing, and a gait disorder resulting in frequent falls. Recently, he has become increasingly withdrawn, anxious, depressed, and distractible, and occasionally he appeared unresponsive. There was no past medical history of meningitis, substance abuse, or toxin exposure. The paternal family was of northern European descent and the maternal family was of non-Jewish Russian and Yugoslavian ancestry. One brother was said to have ataxia and a bipolar mood disorder.

Examination

He was withdrawn and slow to respond to tests of cognitive function. He made errors on tests of attention, calculation, and recall. He had a mixed spastic-ataxic dysarthria. There was moderate, asymmetric dysdiadochokinesia and dysmetria of the upper and lower limbs, and gait was ataxic. Appendicular spasticity, hyperreflexia, and a right Babinski response were present. Cranial nerve function, sensory examination findings, and strength were normal. There were no Kayser-Fleischer rings.

Investigations

Magnetic resonance imaging studies showed marked cerebellar and brainstem atrophy and a posterior fossa cyst (Figure). Studies for spinocerebellar ataxia types 1, 2, 3, 6, and 8 and Friedreich's ataxia were negative. Test results for vitamin B_{12} metabolism, VDRL, ceruloplasmin, thyroid-stimulating hormone, human immunodeficiency virus, and vitamin E deficiency were normal, as were results of cerebrospinal fluid analysis and electroencephalography. Anti-gliadin antibodies were weakly positive.

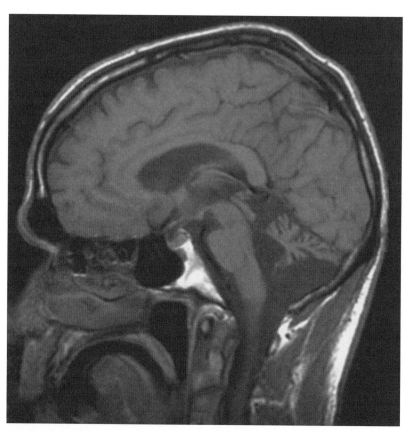

FIGURE. Sagittal magnetic resonance imaging scan demonstrating marked cerebellar and moderate brainstem atrophy.

Commentary by Dr. James H. Bower

The patient's total leukocyte hexosaminidase activity was slightly reduced at 14.5 U/g protein (normal, 16.4-36.2 U/g protein), but percent A was only 5% (normal, 63%-75%). This finding confirmed the diagnosis of GM$_2$ gangliosidosis (adult-onset Tay-Sachs disease). The diagnosis was suspected because the disorder was slowly progressive, spanning more than two decades, with features of cognitive, behavioral, extrapyramidal, pyramidal, and cerebellar dysfunction, and demonstrated cerebellar and brainstem atrophy.

GM$_2$ gangliosidoses are a group of autosomal recessive disorders that result from the accumulation of GM$_2$ ganglioside in neuronal lysosomes. The β-hexosaminidase enzyme cleaves the *N*-acetylgalactosamine moiety from the GM$_2$ ganglioside. Deficiency of this enzyme or its cofactor, the GM$_2$ activator protein, leads to the accumulation of GM$_2$ ganglioside.

β-Hexosaminidase A consists of α and β subunits, whereas β-hexosaminidase B consists of β subunits only. The α subunit is encoded on chromosome 15. More than 75 identified mutations of this gene result in the deficiency of β-hexosaminidase A. The β subunit is encoded on chromosome 5, and 14 identified mutations of this gene result in the deficiency of β-hexosaminidase A and β-hexosaminidase B. Other mutations have been identified in the GM$_2$ activator protein, leading to more than 100 mutations that can cause the accumulation of GM$_2$ ganglioside in lysosomes.

Tay-Sachs disease is an infantile encephalopathy that usually affects the Ashkenazi Jewish population. It is caused by the absence of β-hexosaminidase A. A clinically similar disease, Sandhoff's disease, is caused by the absence of β-hexosaminidase A and β-hexosaminidase B. Since the identification of Tays-Sachs disease and Sandhoff's disease, however, it has been recognized that late juvenile and adult-onset GM$_2$ gangliosidoses also exist and result from only partial enzyme deficiencies.

Adult-onset GM$_2$ gangliosidoses usually present in the first through third decades of life with a varied phenotypic spectrum. Atypical spinocerebellar ataxia, atypical motor neuron disease, and atypical psychosis are the three most common presentations.

Atypical spinocerebellar ataxia with spasticity, dysarthria, and muscle atrophy has been reported in some families. Upper and lower motor neuron findings, dementia, and psychosis may also be present.

Patients may present with motor neuron disease—weakness, cramps, proximal muscle wasting, hyperreflexia, and extensor plantar responses. Ataxia or psychosis may appear later.

Psychosis has been reported in up to one-half of all patients with adult-onset GM_2 gangliosidosis. A mood disorder (either depression or mania or both) has been reported in up to 40% of patients. Phenothiazines and tricyclic antidepressants may worsen the condition because they may inhibit the activity of lysosomal enzymes and thus increase lipidosis.

Other reported clinical features include dystonia, dementia, choreoathetosis, and peripheral neuropathy. Computed tomographic and magnetic resonance imaging scans show cerebellar atrophy and sometimes cerebral atrophy. Rectal biopsy specimens can show the typical membranous cytoplasmic bodies in swollen ganglion cells.

The measurement of β-hexosaminidase A activity is a relatively easy laboratory test to perform to help make the diagnosis. Although only three mutations account for 98% of the mutations that lead to Tay-Sachs disease in the Ashkenazi Jewish population, the numerous mutations that cause the disease in other populations make routine genetic testing in these populations impractical.

Treatment has been unsuccessful. Attempts at enzyme infusion, substrate depletion, bone marrow transplantation, and gene therapy are continuing.

REFERENCE

Federico A, Palmeri S, Malandrini A, *et al*. The clinical aspects of adult hexosaminidase deficiencies. *Dev Neurosci* 1991;**13**:280-7.

History

A 48-year-old man with a known history of pancreatic cancer presented with a 1-week history of severe, continuous pain in the right suboccipital region. The pain radiated to the ipsilateral frontotemporal region and was exacerbated by neck flexion and rotation of the head to the left. One week after the onset of head pain, slurred speech developed. The patient said he had no other neurologic complaints.

Examination

On examination, he held his neck stiffly and had marked tenderness to palpation over the right occipital region. The tongue deviated to the right when protruded. Neurologic examination findings were otherwise normal.

Investigations

Unenhanced T_1-weighted magnetic resonance images of the base of the skull demonstrated a region of abnormal signal intensity involving the right occipital condyle (Figure). After contrast administration, pathologic enhancement of the lesion and adjacent soft tissues was observed. Pain control was achieved with radiotherapy to the skull base.

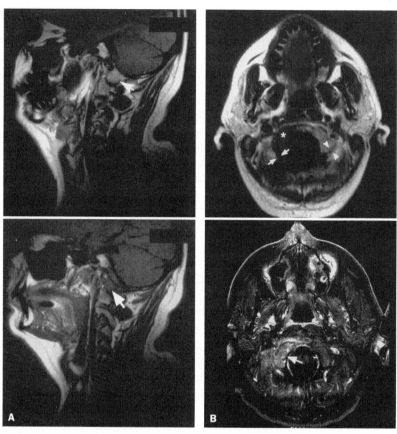

FIGURE. *A, Top,* Sagittal unenhanced T$_1$-weighted magnetic resonance image (MRI) demonstrating the normal appearance of the left occipital condyle (*arrow*). *Bottom,* Sagittal unenhanced T$_1$-weighted MRI demonstrating replacement of the normal marrow by hypointense tissue (*arrow*). *B, Top,* Axial T$_1$-weighted MRI demonstrating the right condyle lesion (*), with abnormal signal extending into the right hypoglossal canal (*arrows*). The left hypoglossal canal (*arrowheads*) is normal. *Bottom,* Axial T$_1$-weighted postcontrast fat saturation MRI demonstrating replacement of the normal marrow within the right occipital condyle (*arrow*). (From Capobianco DJ, Brazis PW, Rubino FA, *et al. Headache* 2002;**42**:142-6. By permission of the American Headache Society.)

Commentary by Dr. Paul W. Brazis

This patient's presentation is an example of the occipital condyle syndrome. This syndrome consists of unilateral pain in the occipital region associated with ipsilateral paresis of cranial nerve XII (the hypoglossal nerve) and is typically due to metastasis to the skull base. Patients with this syndrome complain of continuous, severe, localized, unilateral occipital pain made worse by neck flexion and often associated with neck stiffness. Rotating the head toward the side of the pain often relieves the discomfort, whereas rotating it to the nonpainful side or palpating the suboccipital area is unbearable. The pain occasionally radiates anteriorly toward the ipsilateral temporal area or eye. About half of the patients complain of dysarthria or dysphagia (or both), specifically related to difficulty moving the tongue. On examination, patients hold their neck stiffly and the occipital area on the involved side is often tender to palpation. The ipsilateral tongue is weak and atrophic and deviates toward the weak side. Inflammation or fracture of the occipital condyle may also cause a unilateral or bilateral palsy of cranial nerve XII associated with occipital pain. Skull metastases to the clivus may also cause a bilateral palsy of cranial nerve XII.

We have reported on 11 patients with the occipital condyle syndrome, and all complained of severe pain in the occipital region. Two patients complained of ipsilateral ear or mastoid pain, two noted associated vertex pain, and two had pain in the frontal region. In all patients, the occipital pain was ipsilateral to the hypoglossal nerve paresis. All patients were mildly dysarthric, and three had dysphagia. In seven patients, the pain in the occipital region preceded hypoglossal nerve paresis by several days to 10 weeks. On examination, tenderness to palpation of the occipital region was noted in all patients. All patients had unilateral hypoglossal nerve paresis. Skull films were abnormal in two of the five patients for whom they were obtained, and tomograms were abnormal in one of two patients. Computed tomography, bone scanning, and magnetic resonance imaging were abnormal in all patients in whom they were performed. Nine patients had a known primary malignancy. The most common malignancies were breast cancer in women (two of three women) and prostate cancer in men (four of eight men). In two patients, occipital condyle syndrome was the initial manifestation of a metastatic lesion. Radiotherapy was the treatment of choice for the occipital region pain.

Occipital condyle syndrome is a rare but stereotypic syndrome. Early detection has important therapeutic implications. Evaluation of the craniovertebral junction with attention to the occipital condyles should be a routine part of all brain and cervical spine radiologic examinations, and the possibility of occipital condyle syndrome should be considered, particularly when patients have persistent occipital pain and a history of cancer.

Cranial nerve XII has a close spatial relation with cranial nerves IX, X, and XI in the posterior cranial fossa and as it leaves the skull in the hypoglossal canal. Although a basilar skull lesion (e.g., tumor or trauma) may involve cranial nerve XII alone, it frequently involves the other lower cranial nerves. Damage to all four of these cranial nerves results in Collet-Sicard syndrome, which consists of paralysis of the ipsilateral trapezius and sternocleidomastoid muscles, paralysis of the ipsilateral vocal cord and pharynx, hemiparalysis of the tongue, loss of taste on the posterior third of the ipsilateral tongue, and hemianesthesia of the palate, pharynx, and larynx. Other palsy syndromes involving multiple lower cranial nerves may occur with lesions in the posterior cranial fossa, skull, retropharyngeal or retrostyloid space, or neck.

Another rare syndrome of clinical concern is the combination of cranial nerve VI (abducens nerve) and cranial nerve XII palsies. This ominous combination may be seen with nasopharyngeal carcinoma (Godtfredsen's syndrome) and clival lesions, especially tumors, three-fourths of which are malignant. Although the combination of a cranial nerve VI palsy with a cranial nerve XII palsy usually localizes the pathologic process to the clivus, lower brainstem lesions and subarachnoid processes (e.g., meningitis) may also cause this unusual combination of cranial nerve palsies.

REFERENCE

Capobianco DJ, Brazis PW, Rubino FA, *et al.* Occipital condyle syndrome. *Headache* 2002;**42**:142-6.

History

A 21-year-old man presented for evaluation and treatment of an intractable seizure disorder. He was 15 months old at seizure onset. Initially, he experienced up to 50 1-minute episodes daily of behavioral arrest and staring. At age 11 years, he developed a different type of clinical event associated with pupillary dilatation and jerking of the right arm or leg, followed by generalized stiffening, pelvic flexion and rocking, and repetitive bilateral leg movements. He often fell during these seizures. At the time of the evaluation, the majority of the six to eight daily seizures occurred during sleep and each was approximately 30 to 45 seconds long. The patient would awaken and, without warning or aura, experience a "convulsion" that often resulted in physical trauma. The parents would be awakened by his seizure activity. The longest seizure-free interval in the past several years was 72 hours. Multiple combinations of antiepileptic medications had failed to decrease the frequency or tendency of the seizure activity. He lived with his parents, was unemployed, and required supervision with bathing. He was the product of a normal pregnancy, but labor was prolonged. At age 2, he had a near-drowning experience that required resuscitation. Paternal cousins had seizure disorders.

Examination

The patient had a mild chronic global static encephalopathy. He appeared sedated because of the antiepileptic drug therapy.

Investigations

A wake and sleep electroencephalogram (EEG) demonstrated mild diffuse slowing without epileptiform discharges. A magnetic resonance imaging (MRI) head seizure protocol was normal. Scalp-recorded ictal EEG monitoring did not show a lateralized or localized seizure pattern. A subtracted peri-ictal single-photon emission computed tomography (SPECT) study coregistered to MRI of the patient's head (subtraction of interictal from ictal SPECT coregistered to three-dimensional MRI [SISCOM]) demonstrated a prominent localized region of cerebral hyperperfusion in the inferior and lateral aspect of the left anterior frontal lobe (Figure). He was considered a candidate for intracranial EEG monitoring and possible focal cortical resection. A subdural grid was placed stereotactically over the dorsal convexity of the left anterior frontal lobe. The patient's characteristic seizure activity was associated with an ictal EEG pattern that was intimately related to the localized SISCOM alteration. The ictal onset zone, as determined with intracranial EEG monitoring, was resected.

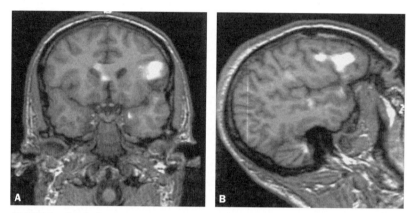

FIGURE. SISCOM study in the, *A*, coronal and, *B*, sagittal (right) planes shows a localized region of cerebral hyperperfusion in the left frontal lobe (see color insert).

Commentary by Dr. Gregory D. Cascino

Pathologic examination of the epileptic brain tissue showed focal cortical dysplasia. The patient has been seizure-free and asymptomatic for more than 5 years after resection. There were no operative complications. The patient's behavior and neurocognitive performance have improved markedly, and he is now employed and does not require supervision. Also, there has been a pronounced reduction in the adverse effects of antiepileptic drug medication. Partial or localization-related epilepsy is the most common seizure disorder. Approximately 90% of the adult incident cases of epilepsy have recurrent and unprovoked partial seizures. An estimated 20% of patients with epilepsy have an intractable seizure disorder, that is, pharmacoresistant seizures that are physically and socially disabling. Coexisting comorbid conditions associated with an intractable seizure disorder often include cognitive impairment, behavioral problems, psychosocial isolation, and the inability to operate a motor vehicle or to be gainfully employed. Patients with medically refractory seizures may also require a supervised living situation or caregiver. A prognostic indicator for an unfavorable response to antiepileptic drug therapy is the identification of a structural lesion as the cause of the seizure disorder. Potential alternative forms of therapy for patients with intractable epilepsy include the use of newer antiepileptic drug medications, surgical treatment, and vagus nerve stimulation.

Epilepsy surgery is safe and effective for selected patients with medically refractory partial epilepsy. For patients with medically refractory seizures, focal resection of the epileptogenic cortex compares favorably with antiepileptic drug treatment and vagus nerve stimulation. Fewer than 10% of patients with intractable seizure disorders are rendered seizure-free with "newer" antiepileptic drug therapy or electronic stimulation. The surgically remediable epileptic syndromes include medial temporal lobe epilepsy and localization-related epilepsy associated with foreign-tissue lesions. Approximately 60% to 80% of favorable surgical candidates are rendered seizure-free after epilepsy surgery. The surgical pathologic lesion most commonly associated with medial temporal lobe epilepsy is mesial temporal sclerosis. Lesional pathology includes tumors, vascular anomalies, and malformations of cortical development. The rationale for operative intervention is to substantially reduce seizure tendency and to allow the person to become a participating and productive member of society.

Focal cortical dysplasia is a malformation of cortical development that may be associated with an early age at seizure onset, cognitive deficits, and medically refractory seizures. MRI, with various degrees of specificity and sensitivity, may demonstrate a localized alteration in patients with a malformation of cortical development, depending on the specific histopathologic features of the lesion. Unremarkable MRI findings, however, do not exclude the presence of focal cortical dysplasia as the cause of a partial seizure disorder.

SISCOM is a recent innovation that may assist in localizing epileptogenic cortex. Functional neuroimaging is particularly important in patients with nonlesional extratemporal seizures. Overall, the outcome of epilepsy surgery for extratemporal seizures is less favorable than for medial temporal lobe epilepsy. Peri-ictal imaging may provide a "target" indicating the likely site of seizure onset and may alter the operative strategy. The use of intracranial EEG monitoring is necessary to map the ictal onset zone and to determine the boundaries of the resection. SISCOM is a reliable indicator of epileptic brain tissue in patients being considered for surgical treatment. The presence of a SISCOM-identified localized region of cerebral hyperperfusion is a predictor of a favorable operative outcome.

REFERENCE

O'Brien TJ, So EL, Mullan BP, *et al.* Subtraction peri-ictal SPECT is predictive of extratemporal epilepsy surgery outcome. *Neurology* 2000;**55**:1668-77.

History

A 67-year-old man was evaluated because he recently noticed mild dysphagia for solids, although he had never noted any facial weakness or trouble drinking through a straw. In 1952, when he was 18 years old, bilateral arm weakness, bilateral scapular winging, and atrophy of the left arm and leg developed after a flu-like illness. Poliomyelitis was diagnosed, but no tests were performed. Except for static atrophy of the left arm and leg, he lived an active life until age 57, when he noted reduced ability to run because of progressive left leg weakness. Gradually progressive, painless atrophy and weakness of affected muscle groups developed, involving primarily the left arm and leg. There was no family history of neuromuscular disease.

Examination

The cranial nerve examination was normal, and no facial weakness or atrophy was found. He had asymmetric, moderate weakness, especially of the proximal muscles of all four limbs, and mild weakness of neck flexors. Severe atrophy of the muscles of the left limbs was most apparent in proximal arm and distal leg muscles. No fasciculations were noted. There was bilateral scapular winging. Deep tendon reflexes were decreased, except for a mildly increased right gastrocnemius reflex. Sensory examination findings were normal. He walked with a left footdrop.

Investigations

Nerve conduction studies showed a low-amplitude right tibial compound muscle action potential. Needle examination demonstrated prominent short-duration, low-amplitude, polyphasic motor unit action potentials in all muscles without fibrillation potentials (Figure). Recruitment was rapid in weak muscles. The creatine kinase level was slightly increased at 387 U/L (normal, <336 U/L). A biopsy specimen from the right vastus lateralis muscle demonstrated changes typical of only denervation atrophy and not of a chronic neurogenic process such as poliomyelitis.

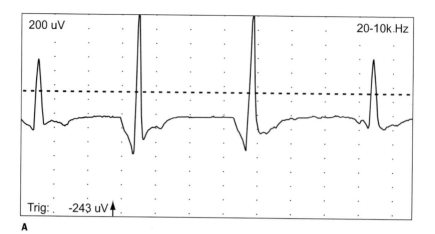

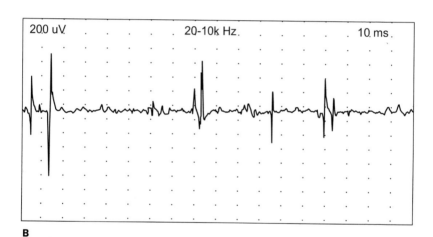

FIGURE. *A,* Normal voluntary motor unit action potentials. *B,* Small, short, myopathic motor units as seen in this patient.

Commentary by Dr. Brian A. Crum

Genetic studies revealed a deletion on chromosome 4q consistent with FSH muscular dystrophy. FSH muscular dystrophy is an autosomal dominant hereditary myopathy caused by deletion of a subtelomeric portion of chromosome band 4q35. The gene product has not been identified, although it is believed that this deletion leads to abnormal expression of another unknown gene or genes. Approximately 25% to 30% of cases are sporadic. The prevalence of the disorder is estimated at 1:20,000. Onset typically occurs by the teenage years, although onset has been reported in patients as old as 75 years. The severity and progression of FSH muscular dystrophy vary widely, but about 20% of patients eventually require wheelchair assistance. The disease may have prolonged periods of stabilization or even complete arrest. Life span is not significantly shortened.

The classic phenotype is that of facial, proximal arm, pelvic, and distal leg weakness. It generally is accepted that FSH muscular dystrophy leads to "descending" weakness, although up to one-half of patients never experience pelvic girdle or leg weakness. Scapulohumeral onset is three times more common than facial onset; however, it may be that symptoms of arm and shoulder weakness first lead to medical evaluation, because at presentation most of the patients with these symptoms already have facial weakness. Other common features include scapular winging, asymmetry, and even congenital absence of individual muscles. The deltoid muscles may be spared. Other features commonly noted include anterior axillary folds and horizontal clavicles. Beevor's sign (the umbilicus moves rostrally on contraction of abdominal muscles with flexion of the neck) may be seen with selective involvement of the lower abdominal muscles. With the advent of genetic testing, atypical presentations of FSH muscular dystrophy have been reported, including facial-sparing myopathy, distal myopathy, asymmetric arm weakness, calf weakness, and proximal weakness simulating limb-girdle muscular dystrophy. Thus, a detailed examination to assess for mild, especially asymmetric, limb weakness, facial weakness, and scapular winging is essential.

Laboratory findings usually include increased levels of creatine kinase; however, after age 55, these levels may decrease or be normal. Electromyographic evaluation shows short-duration, low-amplitude motor units with rapid recruitment. The severity of the findings may vary between muscles and even between different sites in the same muscle. As in chronic myopathies, larger motor units may be seen. Fibrillation potentials may be sparse or prominent. Muscle biopsy specimens demonstrate myopathic changes, with central nuclei, fiber necrosis, variation in fiber diameter, and an increase in perimysial and endomysial connective tissue. Inflammatory infiltrates may be present in the perivascular areas of the endomysium and perimysium. The occurrence of these infiltrates may be genetically determined because they are either present or absent in a given family.

Other systemic manifestations are rare. Deafness is uncommon, although subclinical hearing loss detected by audiometry is not. Coat's disease is a retinal vascular disorder that, although uncommon, may be present, typically in association with severe childhood FSH muscular dystrophy. Exudative leakage from damaged endothelial cells in small retinal blood vessels can threaten vision. Cardiac conduction defects are exceedingly rare. Mental retardation has been associated with FSH muscular dystrophy, but a definite relationship has not been established.

No effective treatment is available for FSH muscular dystrophy. Inflammatory changes may be seen in muscle biopsy specimens; however, the results of a clinical trial of prednisone therapy in FSH muscular dystrophy were negative. A clinical trial of albuterol found an increase in grip strength and lean body mass in the treatment group but no significant improvement in overall muscle strength. Other treatment measures such as scapular fixation and ankle-foot orthoses have a role in symptomatic treatment.

REFERENCE

Felice KJ, Moore SA. Unusual clinical presentations in patients harboring the fascioscapulohumeral dystrophy 4q35 deletion. *Muscle Nerve* 2001;**24**:352-6.

History

Over a 1-year period, a 36-year-old man developed paresthesias of the feet, hypertension, drenching sweats, slurred speech, intermittent hallucinations, severe insomnia, and somniloquy ("like telephone conversations at work"). He had a weight loss of 100 lb despite a good appetite.

Examination

During neurologic examination, he was inattentive and appeared to be experiencing visual hallucinations. Episodes of hyperhydrosis followed by piloerection were observed. His speech was dysarthric. Diffuse myoclonic jerks and continuous involuntary movements characterized as myokymia were seen in major muscle groups.

Investigations

The results of routine biochemical and hematologic studies and two cerebrospinal fluid (CSF) examinations were normal, aside from an increased protein level (70 mg/dL; normal, 14-45 mg/dL) in the CSF.

Antibodies were detected to voltage-gated potassium channels (1,360 pmol/L), GAD65 (0.17 nmol/L; normal, <0.02 nmol/L), and acetylcholine receptor protein binding (0.04 nmol/L; normal, <0.02 nmol/L). Electroencephalography showed diffuse nonspecific slow wave abnormalities. Electromyography (EMG) demonstrated fasciculation potentials, multiplets, and occasional neuromyotonic discharges (Figure). Overnight polysomnography did not demonstrate sleep spindles, K complexes, or neurophysiologic features of sleep. Autonomic testing documented autonomic impairment in addition to autonomic hyperactivity. Computed tomography (CT) of the chest demonstrated a mediastinal mass.

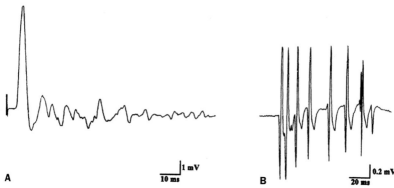

FIGURE. *A*, Peroneal motor response. Stimulation at ankle produced a normal compound muscle action potential, followed by irregular afterdischarges. *B*, Needle electromyography from the medial gastrocnemius muscle shows spontaneous short multiplets with high intraburst frequency (50-150 Hz) consistent with neuromyotonia. (From Josephs KA, Vernino S, Silber MH, *et al*. *Arch Neurol* (in press). By permission of the American Medical Association.)

Commentary by Dr. Keith A. Josephs

Morvan's syndrome, or chorée fibrillaire de Morvan, is characterized by peripheral nerve hyperexcitability, dysautonomia, insomnia, and fluctuating delirium. Typical presenting signs and symptoms include muscle twitching, hyperhydrosis, insomnia, fluctuating cognition, and limb paresthesias. The precise pathophysiologic mechanism of the syndrome is not known, but recent studies support the concept that Morvan's syndrome is an autoimmune or paraneoplastic disorder. Associations with myasthenia gravis, thymoma, and small cell lung cancer have been demonstrated. CT demonstrated that the patient had a malignant thymoma.

Two key features of Morvan's syndrome are 1) spontaneous muscle fiber activity with fasciculation, multiplets, and myokymic and neuromyotonic discharges seen on EMG and 2) serum antibodies specific for neuronal voltage-gated potassium channels. Other laboratory and imaging findings usually are not notably abnormal, but they may aid with the differential diagnosis. Typically, magnetic resonance imaging (MRI), hexamethylpropyleneamine oxime single photon computer emission tomographic, and fluorodeoxyglucose F 18 positron emission tomographic (PET) findings are normal and can help differentiate Morvan's syndrome from limbic encephalitis and fatal familial insomnia. In the latter two conditions, MRI and PET scans are usually abnormal.

Dysautonomia is a prominent feature of Morvan's syndrome. Patients may complain of itching, palmoplantar erythema, and excess sweating. Hypertension and tachycardia are also common. These features of dysautonomia most likely result from peripheral autonomic and sudomotor nerve dysfunction. Insomnia in Morvan's syndrome may be due to interruption of thalamolimbic circuitry.

Therapy should involve treatment of any associated malignancy, followed by either plasma exchange or intravenous administration of gamma globulin. Addition of immunomodulating therapies, including corticosteroids, azathioprine, or cyclophosphamide, may be required for long-term immunosuppression. Alleviating the insomnia is important and, in some cases, may require the use of opioids.

A definitive diagnosis of Morvan's syndrome should be reserved for patients who have at least four cardinal features: clinical myokymia, dysautonomia, insomnia, and fluctuating encephalopathy with vivid hallucinations. Confirmation of Morvan's syndrome requires evidence of spontaneous EMG discharges (neuromyotonia or myokymia) and antibodies to voltage-gated potassium channels.

REFERENCE

Josephs KA, Vernino S, Silber MH, *et al*. Neurophysiologic characterization of Morvan's syndrome. *Arch Neurol* (in press).

History

A 55-year-old woman presented with an 8-year history of a pain disorder. At onset, the pain was a sudden, constant burning sensation that involved an area the size of a U.S. $1 coin (about 2.5 cm) in the right groin. She had no aggravating or relieving factors and no allodynia. Three years after the onset of pain, she noted the sudden onset of "an electrical current" sensation involving the medial aspect of the left leg. The burning groin pain fluctuated, and later both sensations improved spontaneously. No functional deficit was apparent. Previous physicians had noted a minor degree of upper motor neuron weakness and left leg hyperreflexia only. Multiple medications and a transcutaneous electrical nerve stimulation unit had failed to help. One year after the spontaneous improvement, the right groin pain recurred in combination with a new symptom of an intense, distressing itching sensation involving the scapular region bilaterally. Multiple medications, including anticonvulsants, antidepressants, and opiate antagonists, failed to help, but a lidocaine transdermal patch controlled the itching.

Examination

Neurologic examination demonstrated hyperreflexia of the left leg, a left Babinski sign, and hypesthesia to pinprick and thermal stimuli in the right leg.

Investigations

Magnetic resonance imaging (MRI) was performed.

Commentary by Dr. Paola Sandroni

MRI demonstrated a 12-mm minimally enhancing intramedullary lesion within the lower aspect of the thoracic cord suggestive of a cavernous angioma (Figure). Itching (or pruritus) is a sensation that generates an urge to scratch the affected area. Itch generally has been considered a form of pain because it can be as distressing as pain. Indeed, itching is conveyed by C fibers, as is pain sensation. No specific itch receptor is known, and the identity of a fiber population specific for itch is still uncertain. This population may be heterogeneous and consist of both itch-specific and polymodal fibers that also convey pain sensation but are exquisitely sensitive to histamine. Intraneural recordings have documented the existence of both fiber types. Exactly where these fibers end peripherally is not known, but most authors think they terminate in both the dermis and epidermis.

The overlap of pain and itch peripherally also occurs, at least partly, centrally. Pain has two main pathways (one conveying highly discriminative information and the other conveying more diffuse sensation), but itch appears to have only one pathway. However, it is extremely difficult to study itch in isolation from pain. The scratch reflex, particularly in animals, supports the existence of a powerful integration center at the level of the spinal cord. It is at this level that the pathways for itch and pain likely diverge, as suggested by the opposite effect of opiates (i.e., with opiates, especially when adminstered intrathecally, pain decreases and itch increases). Otherwise, the same neurotransmitters that modulate pain can also modulate itch, particularly serotonin.

Although the gate control theory was proposed to explain the modulation of pain sensation, it also applies to itch. The activation of large fibers by scratching is a powerful suppressor of itch. However, activation of thinly myelinated and unmyelinated fibers by cold, heat, and pain also can suppress itch, albeit transiently. Itch and pain almost never coexist in the same area; itch often precedes pain or, less commonly, alternates with it.

In a positron emission tomographic study to identify the topographic representation of itch at the level of the cerebral cortex, mainly premotor areas were activated, suggesting that the study documented the basis of the "urge to scratch." The cingulate cortex also was activated, suggesting the engagement of motivational-emotional and possibly autonomic systems in a reaction to the unpleasant itching experience. The activation of these systems may explain the curious need to scratch while watching someone else do so.

Itch is associated most often with skin conditions, but it is not uncommonly associated with peripheral neuropathies. The few reports of itch caused by a central nervous system lesion included mainly demyelinating disorders or vascular injuries. In these conditions, itching usually is perceived in an area of sensory deficit, suggesting itch has a somatotopic distribution similar to that of the impaired modalities.

The treatment of neuropathic itch is similar to that of neuropathic pain and includes such medications as serotonin-modulating agents, anticonvulsants, antidepressants, and capsaicin. Also, antihistamine agents and opiate antagonists (naltrexone) can be effective. The treatment of neuropathic itch with lidocaine has not been reported, although this agent is helpful in non-neuropathic itch. Because a lidocaine patch is effective in treating neuralgic syndromes (particularly postherpetic neuralgia, which also can manifest with intense itching), it would be expected that lidocaine would be helpful in treating neuropathic itch.

Although little information is available about the management of central neuropathic itch, one would suspect it would be as challenging to manage as a central pain syndrome. The interesting aspect of the case presented here is the central origin of the symptoms, which usually implicates suppression of inhibitory circuits or spontaneous firing of deafferented neurons (or both). Thus, one would not predict a good response to treatment with a topical peripheral agent. The relief provided by the lidocaine patch suggests that peripheral input is critical in somehow modulating the activity of altered central pathways.

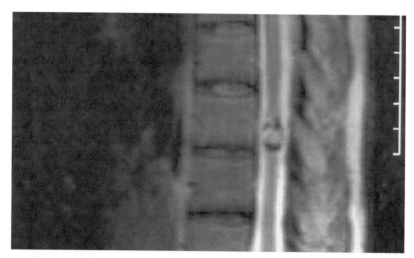

FIGURE. Sagittal T$_2$-weighted image of the thoracic spinal cord showing a peripheral rim of hemosiderin and central zone of increased T$_2$ signal consistent with a cavernous hemangioma. The lesion was enhanced slightly after the administration of gadolinium.

REFERENCE

Sandroni P. Central neuropathic itch: a new treatment option? *Neurology* 2002;**59**:778-9.

History

A 59-year-old man presented with a 6-year history of progressive leg weakness. He needed to interrupt his exercise to sit because his legs felt "like spaghetti." A neurologist diagnosed chronic inflammatory demyelinating polyradiculoneuropathy (CIDP). He received 46 plasma-exchange treatments with apparent partial benefit. However, his condition worsened. Subsequently, he received a brief course of intravenous immunoglobulin and long-term treatment with prednisone in combination with several immunosuppressive drugs, including cyclophosphamide, azathioprine, mycophenolate mofetil, and tacrolimus. Despite treatment, his condition worsened, and he recently noted numbness in the soles of his feet, bladder hesitancy, constipation, and impotence.

Examination

The patient required a cane to ambulate, and he was unable to walk on heels or toes. Neurologic examination demonstrated moderate weakness of ankle dorsiflexors and plantar flexors and mild distal sensory loss affecting light touch, joint position, and vibration sense in the feet and impairment of pin sensation over the feet and sacral area. Deep tendon reflexes were absent in the lower extremities. Muscle strength and sensation were normal in the upper extremities.

Investigations

Hematologic and biochemical tests, the erythrocyte sedimentation rate, and tests for vitamin B_{12}, human immunodeficiency virus, Lyme disease, monoclonal proteins, hepatitis, and human T-cell leukemia viruses I/II were normal. Electromyography (EMG) showed chronic, severe mid-thoracic through sacral radiculopathies on the right without evidence of diffuse polyradiculoneuropathy. Cerebrospinal fluid analysis demonstrated only an elevated protein level (twice normal) and one oligoclonal band. Spinal magnetic resonance imaging (MRI) showed diffuse thickening and enhancement of the lumbosacral nerve roots and a thickened conus medullaris. The results of sural nerve and muscle biopsies and spinal angiography performed elsewhere were unrevealing. Repeat spinal MRI demonstrated enlargement with enhancement of the caudal 4 cm of the spinal cord and conus medullaris, with slight contrast enhancement in the cauda equina.

Commentary by Drs. Guillermo A. Suarez and William E. Krauss

Spinal cord and nerve root biopsy specimens showed changes consistent with a vascular malformation. A second spinal angiographic study was performed, and at a second operation, a right T7 SDAVF was obliterated. SDAVF is a rare and treatable cause of myelopathy. The patient presented here had suggestive, evolving MRI findings with abnormal T_2-signal changes involving the lower thoracic spinal cord and conus medullaris (Figure). However, abnormal vasculature was not seen on several studies and was documented with certainty only during a second spinal angiographic study and with spinal cord biopsy. These findings underscore the difficulty in making the diagnosis of SDAVF and the importance of including SDAVFs in the differential diagnosis of myelopathy and lower motor neuron syndromes, particularly those involving the lower thoracic spinal cord and conus medullaris. Several atypical features led to reconsideration of the original referring diagnosis of CIDP. These included 1) predominant involvement of the lower extremities, 2) electrodiagnostic features showing a thoracolumbar polyradiculopathy without multifocal conduction slowing, conduction block, or temporal dispersion, 3) abnormal MRI findings, with enlargement and enhancement of the caudal thoracic spinal cord and conus medullaris, and 4) lack of definite improvement after prolonged treatment with several immunomodulatory agents.

SDAVF typically presents in the early 60s and has a male predominance. Diagnosis is often delayed. Patients describe lower extremity weakness, leg fatigue, and lower extremity or perineal numbness or burning pain as the initial manifestations. Symptoms are asymmetric in up to one-half of patients. Leg weakness (sometimes with low back pain) while maintaining an erect posture or exercise intolerance is seen in many patients. Symptoms worsen with standing and improve with rest. Upper extremities are involved in only a small proportion of cases (e.g., SDAVFs at the foramen magnum or petrous ridge). Symptoms of sphincter dysfunction are usually a late manifestation. In order of frequency, the following initial symptoms predominate: lower extremity weakness, lower extremity fatigue, and lower extremity or perineal numbness (or both). Upper and lower motor neuron signs are found in 70% of patients and lower motor neuron signs alone occur in about 30%. Symptoms progress slowly or with stepwise worsening until the diagnosis and treatment are established. Occasional subacute exacerbations have been described.

EMG localizes the abnormality to the spinal nerve roots or anterior horn cells and excludes other conditions. EMG findings may be entirely normal in the early stages of the disease or show segmental nerve root (polyradiculopathy) or anterior horn cell involvement, especially in the thoracolumbar region. Neuroimaging of the spinal cord with MRI or computed tomographic (CT) myelography demonstrates intramedullary T_2-signal abnormalities, especially in the lower thoracic spinal cord and conus medullaris, associated with abnormal dorsal vessels. CT myelography with prone and supine images reveals dilated vessels on the dorsal surface of the spinal cord. SDAVFs are confirmed and localized by spinal angiography. MRI of the entire spinal cord is the initial diagnostic method of choice because it is noninvasive and allows visualization of the spinal cord and adjacent structures, with high definition. Spinal magnetic resonance angiography can sometimes localize the fistula, directing and streamlining subsequent angiography.

The fistula results from an abnormal connection between a dural artery and a radiculomedullary vein in the dura mater near a nerve root, usually in the thoracolumbar region. The suspected pathogenesis involves venous hypertension leading to neuronal and central nervous system damage. The cause of SDAVFs is unknown, but they are thought to be acquired.

Currently, there are two treatments. Endovascular embolization of acrylic material has a good success rate in experienced centers but is associated with a higher complication rate, a higher rate of treatment failure, and a higher recurrence rate than microsurgical obliteration. We favor surgical intradural disconnection of the fistula because the procedure directly reverses the pathophysiologic mechanism by isolating and disconnecting the proximal draining vein of the SDAVF. In experienced hands, surgery has very low failure and complication rates.

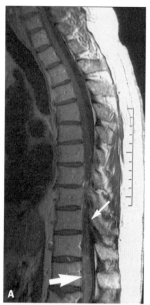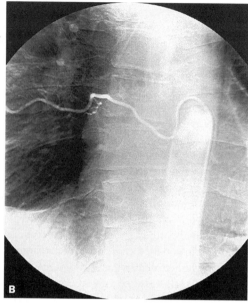

FIGURE. *A*, T$_1$-weighted sagittal image with contrast showing enlargement and abnormal enhancement of the distal thoracic spinal cord and conus medullaris (*thick arrow*). *Thin arrow*, Dilated vessels on posterior surface of the spinal cord. *B*, Spinal angiogram demonstrating a dural arteriovenous fistula at T7 on the right.

REFERENCE

Atkinson JLD, Miller GM, Krauss WE, *et al.* Clinical and radiographic features of dural arteriovenous fistula, a treatable cause of myelopathy. *Mayo Clin Proc* 2001;**76**:1120-30.

History

A 59-year-old man developed paresthesias of both feet. This was followed within weeks by early satiety, postprandial vomiting of undigested
food, and reduced frequency of bowel movements. He became completely unable to eat and lost 60 lb. A J-tube was placed. He had a 40 pack-
year cigarette habit, but extensive studies for malignancy were negative.
In the subsequent weeks, dry mouth, orthostatic hypotension, lower
extremity loss of sweating, and impotence developed. Medical therapy
failed to improve the gastrointestinal dysmotility. Eleven months into
the illness, refractory simple partial and secondary generalized seizures
developed, with postical aphasia, headaches, short-term memory loss,
depression, and night sweats. He was treated with plasma exchange
and oral cyclophosphamide. His gastrointestinal symptoms improved
markedly, and he was able to resume a normal diet. His seizures became
easier to control. He was able to return to work part time on his farm.

Examination

The pupillary light reflex was normal. Other findings included a mild
reduction in short-term memory and asymmetric loss of pin and temperature sensations in a stocking distribution. His feet were dry.
Measurement of blood pressure with the patient standing revealed
orthostatic hypotension.

Investigations

Autonomic studies documented orthostatic hypotension and a blunted
heart rate response to a Valsalva maneuver. Sweating was reduced in the
legs. Gastroparesis and delayed small-bowel transit time were demonstrated. At presentation, serum type 1 antineuronal nuclear autoantibody
(ANNA-1) was detected (1:15,360). Cranial magnetic resonance imaging
(MRI) showed mild atrophy and increased fluid attenuation inversion
recovery (FLAIR) signal in the left mesial temporal, insular, and opercular
cortices (Figure). The results of an exploratory mediastinoscopy and a
video-assisted thoracic surgery procedure were negative. Computed
tomographic (CT) scans of the chest at 3-month intervals and positron
emission tomographic (PET) scans were uninformative. Thirty months
after the onset of symptoms, chest CT demonstrated a small lesion in the
right upper lobe that remained stable for several months. Eight months
later, this lesion had enlarged and a right upper lobectomy was performed.

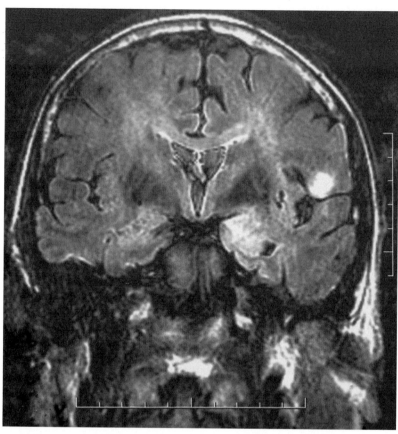

FIGURE. Coronal FLAIR magnetic resonance image demonstrating a non-enhancing signal abnormality in the left amygdala and inferior frontal cortex, with associated mesial temporal atrophy.

Commentary by Dr. Steven Vernino

Neurologic paraneoplastic syndromes are rare but severe neuroim-munologic complications of malignancy. The tumors most commonly associated with these syndromes are small cell lung carcinoma, ovarian carcinoma, breast carcinoma, and thymoma. At surgery, a 1.0 x 1.0 x 1.0-cm grade 3 (of 4) squamous cell carcinoma was identified. These syndromes usually have a subacute onset and a relentlessly progressive clinical course leading to profound morbidity. Typically, the neurologic presentation antedates the diagnosis of malignancy, and the cancer, when found, tends to be localized and responsive to treatment. Clinical manifestations can be quite varied and multifocal in the nervous system. Several distinct clinical syndromes are recognized, including sensory neuronopathy, cerebellar degeneration, limbic encephalitis, brainstem encephalitis, and opsoclonus-myoclonus. Many patients, however, have a combination of symptoms that do not fit neatly into a single syndromic classification. The MRI findings in this patient are typical of paraneoplastic limbic encephalitis. Extratemporal radiographic involvement, particularly of the insular cortex, is not uncommon.

Paraneoplastic limbic encephalitis affects the mesial temporal lobe and mesial limbic structures (cingulate gyrus, orbitofrontal cortex, and mamillary bodies), resulting in the typical triad of memory impairment, temporal lobe seizures, and psychiatric symptoms (including dramatic personality changes, hallucinations, or depression). Small cell carcinoma of the lung is the most commonly associated neoplasm, but other types of cancer have been identified.

Autonomic neuropathy can occur as a remote effect of malignancy, although paraneoplastic nerve disorders also manifest as sensorimotor neuropathy, polyradiculoneuropathy, or sensory neuronopathy. Para-neoplastic autonomic neuropathy can present as subacute severe pandysautonomia but more frequently takes the form of severe gastrointestinal dysmotility (gastroparesis or intestinal pseudo-obstruction). Pathologically, paraneoplastic dysmotility has been associated with an inflammatory destructive process affecting myenteric ganglia of the gut.

Several neuronal autoantibodies have been reported as markers of paraneoplastic limbic encephalitis or paraneoplastic dysautonomia, including ANNA-1 (also known as "anti-Hu"), amphiphysin-IgG, col-lapsin response-mediator protein-5 (CRMP-5)-IgG, parietal cell anitbody-2

(PCA-2), ANNA-3, and "anti-Ma." No clear pathogenic relation has been established between any of these specific antibodies and a particular neurologic syndrome. Despite a typical clinical course and the detection of small cell lung carcinoma, a small proportion of patients with paraneoplastic neurologic disorders lack any of the currently recognized autoantibody markers. Most of the autoantibodies are highly predictive of specific neoplasms. For example, small cell lung carcinoma is found in more than 80% of patients who are seropositive for ANNA-1. Seropositivity for ANNA-1 should prompt a careful evaluation for an underlying small cell lung carcinoma, even if routine imaging studies are negative. PET imaging of the chest is proving to be more sensitive than CT.

Paraneoplastic neurologic symptoms usually precede the diagnosis of cancer, and, as in the case presented here, the diagnosis of malignancy may be delayed for many years. In some cases, a small focus of malignancy is found only at autopsy.

Despite evidence of an autoimmune pathogenesis of these disorders, immunomodulatory treatment generally has been regarded as ineffective. Treatment of the underlying malignancy is considered the mainstay of treatment for these disorders. In some cases, immunomodulatory treatment with high doses of corticosteroids, plasma exchange, intravenous immunoglobulin, or conventional immunosuppressive agents (e.g., cyclophosphamide) offers a reasonable chance of arresting neurologic progression. Treatment is most likely to benefit patients who are not severely disabled, probably because they have less permanent neuronal loss and therefore a better substrate for rehabilitation and for restoration of function through plasticity. Patients without active malignancy need close oncologic follow-up because immunosuppressive treatment has the potential to impair immune surveillance for malignancy.

The patient presented here received cyclophosphamide for 9 months and since then has had sustained clinical and radiographic improvement. He has residual memory deficit and requires anticonvulsant therapy.

REFERENCE

Lucchinetti CF, Kimmel DW, Lennon VA. Paraneoplastic and oncologic profiles of patients seropositive for type 1 antineuronal nuclear autoantibodies. *Neurology* 1998;**50**:652-7.

History

A 60-year-old man developed intermittent diplopia, followed by progressive nausea, vomiting, anorexia, and a severe progressive four-limb and gait ataxia. Within 1 year he was unable to stand or walk without assistance.

Examination

His eye movements were ataxic, and he had a mixed, moderately severe ataxic and spastic dysarthria with a mild flaccid component. Neurologic examination documented severe appendicular and truncal ataxia with a high-amplitude terminal tremor, weakness in the right leg, normal sensory findings, and bilateral Babinski responses.

Investigations

Extensive hematologic, biochemical, and immunologic studies (including paraneoplastic serologic tests) were negative. Tests for syphilis, Lyme disease, and human immunodeficiency virus were normal. A small monoclonal IgG kappa peak (0.2 g/dL) was identified on serum protein electrophoresis. Magnetic resonance imaging (MRI) of the brain showed a bilaterally symmetric distribution of T_2-signal change, with patchy enhancement of the entire brainstem and the pial surface near the cerebral peduncles (Figure). Cerebrospinal fluid studies showed one nucleated cell; the protein and glucose levels were normal.

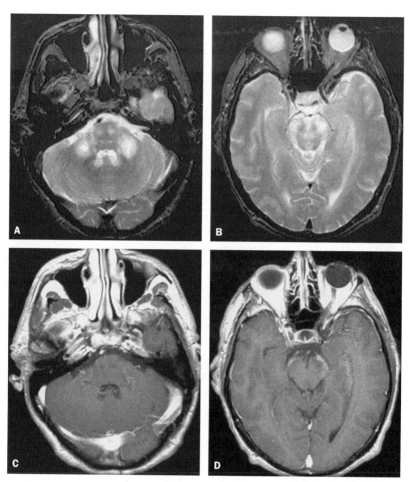

FIGURE. *A* and *B*, Patchy, approximately symmetric areas of T$_2$-signal abnormality in the pons, middle cerebellar peduncles, and midbrain. *C* and *D*, Patchy, somewhat symmetric enhancement of the brainstem near the cerebral peduncle.

Commentary by Dr. David W. Kimmel

Whipple's disease was diagnosed when the polymerase chain reaction (PCR) of the cerebrospinal fluid and small-bowel biopsy specimen were positive for *Tropheryma whippelii*. Whipple's disease is caused by a periodic acid-Schiff (PAS)-positive, weakly gram-positive rod-shaped bacillus, *Tropheryma whippelii*, an organism difficult to cultivate in vitro. Humans are the only natural host for the disease. The infection may be acquired by ingestion. PCR is valuable as a diagnostic tool. An immunohistochemical assay may be helpful.

The mean age at diagnosis is about 50 years, but cases in children and octogenarians have been reported. Predominantly, men are affected (80% of cases). The most common presenting symptoms are diarrhea, abdominal pain, weight loss, fever, and arthritis. Isolated neurologic symptoms are the presenting symptoms in only 5% of patients. Diarrhea and weight loss are present in more than 75% of patients. Other common systemic manifestations include arthralgia, abdominal pain, fever, lymphadenopathy, skin darkening, and steatorrhea. Anemia, increased erythrocyte sedimentation rate, and hypoalbuminemia are common laboratory findings. Occasionally, after antibiotic treatment for systemic disease, patients have relapse with only neurologic involvement.

A multifocal process with small granuloma formation (PAS-positive-staining macrophages surrounded by reactive astrocytes) is seen predominantly in the gray matter (cerebral cortex, hypothalamus, and brainstem). The process may extend into the subarachnoid space.

Neurologic manifestations vary. The combination of cognitive changes, oculomotor abnormalities, myoclonus, and hypothalamic dysfunction is a classic finding. Headache, hemiparesis, and ataxia have all been observed in 10% to 30% of patients. Subacute or chronic cognitive changes, including dementia, isolated memory loss, somnolence, apathy, depression, anxiety, and aphasia, have been reported in at least 50% of patients with neurologic involvement. Early in the illness, these symptoms can be mistaken for a psychiatric disorder.

From 40% to 50% of patients have oculomotor abnormalities, most commonly supranuclear gaze palsy. Vertical involvement is more common than horizontal. Ataxic eye movements and nystagmus are common. Isolated oculomotor palsy is rare. Internuclear ophthalmoplegia has been reported, as have uveitis, retinitis, keratitis, and optic neuropathy.

Perhaps the most interesting disorder is oculomasticatory myorhythmia (OMM), characterized by 1/s pendular horizontal convergent-divergent oscillations of the eyes synchronous with involuntary contractions of masticatory muscles. OMM, specific for Whipple's disease, occurs in only 10% to 20% of patients with neurologic involvement. Oculo-facial-skeletal myorhythmia is a similar disorder, with movements that also involve facial, neck, or extremity muscles. Isolated myoclonus may occur. Hypothalamic involvement resulting in sleep disturbance, polydipsia, and eating disorders has been reported. The triad of dementia, ophthalmoplegia, and myoclonus occurs in 10% of patients.

MRI findings include multiple (occasionally single) T_2-signal lesions that may enhance. Larger lesions may be associated with edema and mass effect. Cerebrospinal fluid analysis usually shows mild to moderate pleocytosis and an increased level of protein. PAS-positive cells are seen occasionally. Electron microscopy may be helpful. PCR of the blood and cerebrospinal fluid appears to be highly specific and sensitive. Often, the diagnosis can be confirmed by analyzing biopsy specimens of the small bowel or lymph nodes with PAS staining, electron microscopy, and PCR.

Treatment involves prolonged administration of antibiotics, although the selection of antibiotics is empirical. Patients may have relapse even after a long course of antibiotic therapy, and occasionally the disease worsens with treatment, suggesting resistance. Relapse is most likely to occur if treatment was with a single antibiotic or with antibiotics that do not cross the blood-brain barrier. Current guidelines recommend an initial course of ceftriaxone or high-dose, intravenously administered penicillin and streptomycin for 2 weeks to 2 months, followed by either trimethoprim-sulfamethoxazole or cefixime for at least 1 to 2 years. PCR may be used to monitor response. Corticosteroids appear to be of no use and may be detrimental. The prognosis depends on the nature and severity of neurologic involvement. Neurologic improvement has been reported in about two-thirds of patients and may be dramatic, but many patients are left with neurologic deficits.

The patient presented here was given ceftriaxone intravenously for 4 weeks and then oral bactrim DS for 4 years. His balance and speech improved gradually and significantly, and the MRI appearance improved. At 4-year follow-up, his dysarthria was mild and he could walk without difficulty, although he could not walk in tandem.

REFERENCE

Marth T, Raoult D. Whipple's disease. *Lancet* 2003;361:239-46.

History

A 39-year-old man presented with an 8-year history of episodic diplopia, progressive dysarthria, dysphagia, and limb and gait clumsiness. He stated that he had not noticed any cognitive or sensory changes or weakness but did need a cane to prevent falls. Throughout the 8 years, he experienced the feeling of a severe tightness that ascended rapidly from his foot to involve one-half of either side of his body. He had multiple episodes of this spell daily, each lasting 15 seconds. During a spell, he could drop an object from the involved hand or lose his balance. Treatment with carbamazepine, 200 mg twice daily, completely prevented these spells. He had abused alcohol and recreational drugs for several years. Three of his several dozen cousins were said to have multiple sclerosis.

Examination

The findings on neurologic examination included ataxic nystagmus, saccadic pursuit, and a moderate spastic-ataxic dysarthria. Also, lower limb spasticity, bilateral extensor toe signs, and mild four-limb and moderate gait ataxia were noted. Motor strength and sensation were normal. Hyperventilation did not evoke a spell.

Investigations

The results of extensive hematologic and biochemical studies, including a peroxisomal panel and tests for syphilis, leukodystrophies, and ceruloplasmin, were normal. Findings on cerebrospinal fluid analysis were entirely normal. Genetic analyses for spinocerebellar ataxia types 1, 2, 3, 6, and 7 and CAG analysis for dentatorubral-pallidoluysian atrophy were negative. Magnetic resonance imaging (MRI) demonstrated marked medullary and moderate cerebellar atrophy (Figure). Areas of contrast enhancement were apparent in the brachium pontis bilaterally. After genetic counseling, a stereotactic brain biopsy was performed.

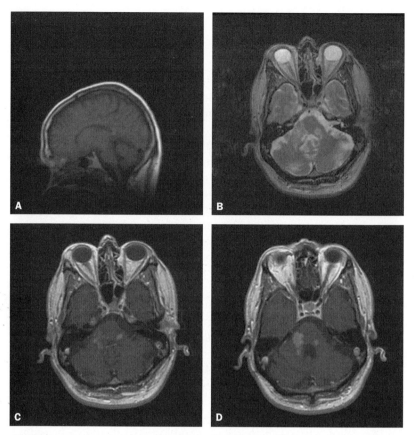

FIGURE. Magnetic resonance images demonstrating *A*, atrophy of the brainstem and cerebellum, *B*, bilateral T$_2$-signal change, and, *C* and *D*, contrast enhancement in the brachium pontis.

Commentary by Dr. John H. Noseworthy

The brain biopsy specimen demonstrated excessive deposition of Rosenthal fibers in the gray and white matter of the middle cerebellar peduncle compatible with adult Alexander's disease.

The infantile form of this central nervous system disorder was first described by Alexander in 1949. The clinical and MRI spectrum of Alexander's disease and its molecular basis have been expanded considerably in recent years. Most cases of the disease are sporadic, but familial cases occur. Infantile (onset before age 2 years) and juvenile forms are more common than the adult form.

Infants usually present with slowing of mental and motor development, macrocephaly, long tract signs, seizures, and hydrocephalus. Death usually occurs within the first decade of life. The typical MRI appearance in infantile Alexander's disease includes widespread white matter changes, predominantly in the frontal lobes; a high signal rim in the periventricular regions on T_1-weighted scans; and changes in the deep gray matter, including the thalami, basal ganglia, and brainstem. Contrast enhancement is common, and widespread demyelination may involve the arcuate, or "U," fibers, sometimes with white matter cavitation.

Disease beginning after age 4 years (juvenile and adult) is considerably more heterogeneous and may progress slowly or remain stable for a prolonged period. In juveniles, the disease may present with spastic weakness, ataxia, and brainstem involvement (including palatal myoclonus, nystagmus, and bulbar and pseudobulbar palsy), usually without cognitive decline. In adults, the disease may mimic multiple sclerosis, with progressive spastic weakness, brainstem syndromes (including bulbar and pseudobulbar palsy, oculomotor abnormalities, neuralgic pain), ataxia, and marked atrophy of the brainstem and cerebellum seen on MRI. Adult Alexander's disease may be discovered incidentally at autopsy, indicating that a mild, nonprogressive type of the disease occurs.

The deposition of Rosenthal fibers in perivascular, subpial, and periventricular regions is the pathologic hallmark of Alexander's disease. Rosenthal fibers consist of intracytoplasmic inclusions in astrocytes of glial fibrillary acidic protein (GFAP), heat shock protein 27, and αβ-crystallin. Both the GFAP and αβ-crystallin genes have been considered candidate genes in Alexander's disease, but no abnormalities in αβ-crystallin genes have been found. A transgenic mouse model of Alexander's disease expressing the human GFAP gene mimics the clinical syndrome of shortened survival and Rosenthal fiber formation, suggesting that Alexander's disease may be a "gain of function" disorder. Recent studies have determined that several nonconservative mutations in the coding region of the GFAP gene are responsible for infantile and juvenile Alexander's disease. Parents of these children have not shown these mutations, suggesting that they are de novo dominant mutations in the GFAP gene. A recent report has confirmed that pathologically proven hereditary adult Alexander's disease also may result from a GFAP gene missense mutation. Further work is needed to determine how often hereditary adult cases represent de novo dominant mutations versus incomplete penetrance or germline mosaicism.

The patient presented here had frequent stereotypic events that were completely responsive to a low dose of carbamazepine. The symptoms were highly reminiscent of paroxysmal spells seen in patients with multiple sclerosis and thought to be caused by ephaptic "crosstalk" between axons at sites of demyelination. This is of interest because of reports of neuralgic pain in other cases of adult Alexander's disease. Of additional interest in relation to the case presented here are reports of sporadic Alexander's disease developing in association with drug and alcohol abuse (and also in association with complex chronic illnesses, including systemic malignancy). Other than supportive care, no definitive treatment is available for this disease. The condition of the patient reported here worsened for 3 years after evaluation, and he died. An autopsy performed elsewhere confirmed the diagnosis.

REFERENCE

Namekawa M, Takiyama Y, Aoki Y, et al. Identification of GFAP gene mutation in hereditary adult-onset Alexander's disease. *Ann Neurol* 2002;**52:**779-85.

History

A 51-year-old man had a 7-year history of urinary hesitancy that did not improve after bladder outlet dilatation and prostatic resection. Five years before the present evaluation, urinary incontinence developed. Within the last 2 years, he has noted progressive impotence, painless lower extremity weakness, and poor balance. He trips easily. Friends at work have commented that he limps. He recently initiated bladder self-catheterization. He reports that he does not have decreased sensation in the feet but does have occasional shooting foot pain, and he has not experienced cognitive decline. His past medical history is unremarkable. He is not of Ashkenazi Jewish heritage, his parents are not consanguineous, and there is no family history of neurologic disease.

Examination

The patient scored 37/38 on the short test of mental status, missing 1 point on recall. He has moderate bilateral weakness of the ankle and toe extensors and slight weakness of the gastrocnemius muscles. Pes cavus is present, and there is slight lower limb spasticity. The knee jerks are increased and the ankle jerks slightly decreased. Neurologic testing demonstrated nonsustained left ankle clonus, bilateral extensor plantar responses, and moderately reduced vibration sense at the toes. He has a steppage and ataxic gait and has more difficulty walking on his heels than on his toes. There is mild lower limb incoordination and slowing of alternating motion rates.

Investigations

The findings of extensive laboratory testing were negative except for a mild increase in the serum level of lactate on three occasions and a twofold increase in creatine kinase. Cerebrospinal fluid examination showed only a slightly elevated protein concentration. The results of nerve conduction and electromyographic studies were consistent with a chronic axonal sensorimotor polyradiculoneuropathy. Neuropsychometric testing revealed mild problems in verbal fluency, visual attention, and executive reasoning and problem-solving abilities. Magnetic resonance imaging demonstrated severe generalized cerebellar and brainstem atrophy, with mild cerebral atrophy (Figure). Multiple, bilateral, nonenhancing focal and confluent areas of increased T_2 signal were present in the periventricular, subcortical, and deep white matter.

Additional T_2-signal abnormality was seen in the internal and external capsules, midbrain, pons, superior cerebellar peduncles, dentate nuclei, and anterior medulla to the level of the cervicomedullary junction, and there was diffuse spinal cord atrophy from C2 to T11. Sural nerve and muscle biopsies were performed.

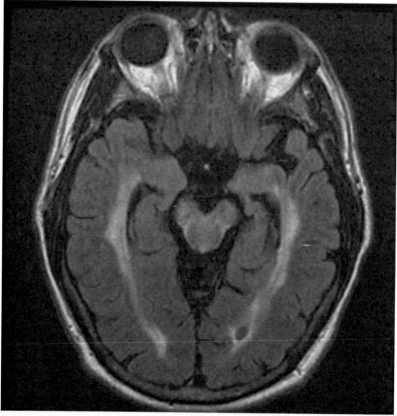

FIGURE. Axial FLAIR image demonstrating diffuse abnormal increased signal within the midbrain and confluent signal abnormality in the periventricular white matter adjacent to the temporal horns of the lateral ventricles. (From Klein CJ, Boes CJ, Chapin JE, *et al. Muscle Nerve* 2004;**29**:323-8. By permission of John Wiley & Sons.)

Commentary by Dr. Christopher J. Boes

The sural nerve specimen demonstrated frequent polyglucosan bodies in axons, and an axillary skin biopsy specimen showed them in the luminal cells of apocrine glands. Muscle biopsy showed diastase-resistant, periodic acid-Schiff (PAS)-positive material in a small population of muscle fibers. Glycogen branching enzyme (GBE) activity from skin fibroblasts was markedly decreased at 178 units (normal, 1,300±390 units). These findings suggested the diagnosis of APBD. APBD is a rare neurologic disorder characterized by progressive upper and lower motor neuron signs, early urinary incontinence, and cognitive impairment. The disease was first described in 1971, and since then, approximately 50 cases have been reported in the English-language literature. Most patients present in the fifth or sixth decade of life with symptoms and signs of myelopathy, peripheral neuropathy, and neurogenic bladder. Weakness and sensory loss typically start in the lower extremities. Approximately 70% of the reported patients have some degree of cognitive impairment, which can become severe later in the course of the disease. The dementia affects cortical and subcortical functions. The symptoms progress over a variable number of years until death. This combination of peripheral nervous system (PNS) and central nervous system (CNS) disease with early sphincter problems is unique. APBD can simulate amyotrophic lateral sclerosis, but the cognitive changes, sphincter involvement, and sensory loss would be unusual for that disease.

Polyglucosan bodies are PAS-positive, diastase-resistant glucose polymers found in the CNS and PNS of patients with APBD as well as in several systemic organs. They occur primarily in neuronal and astrocytic processes. They also can be seen in the CNS and PNS of 1) patients with glycogen storage disease type IV, 2) patients with progressive myoclonic epilepsy (Lafora bodies), and 3) normal subjects (corpora amylacea). CNS polyglucosan bodies are present as "Bielschowsky bodies" in the syndrome of double athetosis. Polyglucosan bodies in sural nerve are nonspecific and can be seen in various clinical disorders, including diabetes mellitus, and with normal aging.

APBD appears to be a heterogeneous condition. Most cases are sporadic, but familial clustering has been reported. In seven Jewish patients with APBD, GBE activity was decreased in leukocytes and peripheral nerve. In these patients, APBD is thought to be an allelic variant of glycogen storage disease type IV, which is a childhood disease caused by deficient GBE activity that typically presents with systemic manifestations. A homozygous mutation (Tyr329Ser) has been considered causative in GBE-deficient APBD patients of Jewish heritage. Several non-Jewish patients with APBD have been reported to have normal GBE activity, and two non-Jewish patients (including this case) have been reported to have low GBE activity. In one of these two patients, two heterozygous mutations (Arg515His, Arg524Gln) were thought to be causative. In the patient presented here, a heterozygous missense alteration (Val160Ile) was found in the GBE gene.

The findings on magnetic resonance imaging (MRI) were consistent with those of previously reported cases of APBD: bilateral, symmetric, nonenhancing areas of signal abnormality in the periventricular and subcortical white matter and diffuse spinal cord atrophy. Unique MRI findings in the patient reported here included T_2-signal hyperintensity in the medullary olives, dentate nuclei, superior cerebellar peduncles, midbrain, and internal and external capsules and prominent vermian atrophy. Nerve conduction and electromyographic studies in APBD generally provide evidence of an axonal sensorimotor peripheral neuropathy, although demyelinating features have also been described.

The diagnosis of probable APBD can be made if a patient has the typical clinical phenotype and an excessive number of polyglucosan bodies in a peripheral nerve biopsy specimen. Axillary skin biopsy specimens can also show polyglucosan bodies. In APBD, the finding of polyglucosan bodies in premortem muscle biopsy specimens is rare and has been reported in only three cases (including this case). Finding GBE deficiency provides a definitive diagnosis in a patient with the typical clinical presentation and sural nerve polyglucosan bodies, but if the GBE level is normal, definitive pathologic diagnosis would await postmortem examination of the brain, spinal cord, and other tissues. There is no established treatment for APBD.

REFERENCE

Klein CJ, Boes CJ, Chapin JE, *et al.* Adult polyglucosan body disease: case description of an expanding genetic and clinical syndrome. *Muscle Nerve* 2004;**29**:323-8.

History

A 53-year-old man had a 2-year history of feeling unsteady when standing. He felt that his legs were shaking and thought he might fall. He preferred to lean against fixed objects such as doorways. His symptoms gradually worsened, and he felt that he had to walk in place while standing still in order to maintain his balance. He had to stop playing tennis because he could no longer stand to receive the serve. In time, he needed to stop shaving while standing and could no longer stand comfortably in line. He felt completely well while sitting or lying down. His past medical history was notable for daytime drowsiness with sleep attacks and cataplexy since age 20.

Examination

The findings on neurologic examination were essentially normal with the following exceptions. While standing, his legs seemed to "shimmer," with rapid muscle contractions visible in the quadriceps muscle. These same contractions were seen when he sat and extended either leg at the knee. No tremor was observed in the upper extremity. Gait was normal.

Investigations

Electrophysiologic recording demonstrated a 14-Hz regular tremor in the quadriceps muscle which was present only while the patient was standing (Figure). It appeared to attenuate when he would "march in place."

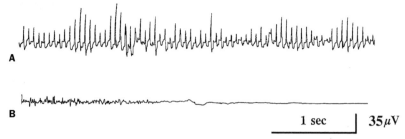

FIGURE. Surface electromyography recording from iliopsoas-hamstring muscle while patient is standing (*A*) and sitting (*B*). Note that the 15-Hz tremor resolves with muscle relaxation.

Commentary by Dr. Ryan J. Uitti

The patient's complaint illustrates the scope of the differential diagnosis of "unsteadiness." Shaking restricted to the legs is an unusual complaint, and unsteadiness does not typically dissipate with walking or movement. Patients with Parkinson's disease usually note tremor or akathisia in the legs only while at rest when sitting or lying. Patients with essential tremor may complain of tremulousness and unsteadiness in the legs with action but typically have accompanying tremor in the arms, head and neck, or voice. In contrast, the worst unsteadiness and shaking in this patient with orthostatic tremor occurred while he was standing in place, as in line at the bank or grocery store. Often, a patient with orthostatic tremor may not report "shaking" but rather a sense of unpleasant, "vibratory" unsteadiness, further contributing to the diagnostic challenge. This patient's history of sleep attacks and cataplexy also suggests a diagnosis of narcolepsy, although this is seemingly unrelated to the chief complaint.

Orthostatic tremor is an unusual disorder that typically involves the legs during standing, hence the term "shaky legs syndrome." When limb muscles are relaxed, the tremulous contractions cease. Similarly, during walking, the sense of tremor dissipates. Patients complain of being unable to stand in one position and report relief with leaning against objects or walking. If patients with orthostatic tremor are asked to support their weight with their arms, similar shaking develops in these limbs. Upon standing, there is often a delay of seconds or minutes before the tremor develops.

"Orthostatic tremor" was first described by Heilman in 1984. The rate of "tremor" is faster than with other forms of tremor, namely 14 to 17 Hz. Because of the speed of the tremor, patients may appear to be vibrating rather than exhibiting gross shaking. Electrophysiologic studies suggest that the tremor is less regular in frequency than in essential tremor or parkinsonism. The tremor is produced by 14- to 17-Hz contractions in agonist-antagonist muscles. Typically, these muscles appear to contract simultaneously (as opposed to the alternating pattern observed in parkinsonism).

The pathogenesis of orthostatic tremor is unknown. Some believe it is a form of essential tremor, whereas others think it is an exaggerated physiologic response to instability or a form of epilepsy. Sharbrough, an emeritus Mayo Clinic electroencephalographer, was the first to note that coincident, fast midline electroencephalographic (EEG) activity (14-17 Hz) may accompany the leg tremors of the same rate. However, fewer than 20% of patients demonstrate these coincident EEG and surface electromyographic findings.

Treatment with clonazepam (0.5-2.0 mg) may be beneficial. Layton, an emeritus Mayo Clinic neurologist, used to keep clonazepam in his desk drawer to confirm the diagnosis and to treat the condition at the same visit. The patient presented here had a positive response to clonazepam treatment and was able to resume all the usual activities that require standing. Other treatments include valproic acid, gabapentin, propranolol, levodopa, and pramipexole. With time (usually decades), some patients develop accompanying gait difficulties, particularly difficulty with gait ignition that may be reminiscent of parkinsonism.

REFERENCE

McManis PG, Sharbrough FW. Orthostatic tremor: clinical and electrophysiologic characteristics. *Muscle Nerve* 1993;**16:**1254-60.

History

A 30-year-old man had a 17-year history of daily headaches. Initially, he had an attack once a month, but for the last 15 years, he had three to five attacks per day (range, 1-12 daily). The headaches occurred during the day or night, awakened him, usually lasted about 30 minutes (15 minutes to 8 hours) and were always on the right side. Severe right supraorbital and hemicranial pain peaked within minutes, often preceded by a 10-minute aura of change in sensation behind his right nostril. Ergotamine would abort 30% of these attacks if taken early. The headaches were associated with one to three episodes of brief loss of consciousness during a 30-minute headache attack. There was no tearing or conjunctival injection. He had bilateral nasal stuffiness, rhinorrhea, nausea, and profound photophobia; alcohol prolonged the attacks. The headaches were often precipitated by exposure to cold air, chocolate, or chewing a pen between his teeth. Multiple medications were tried but failed to provide benefit. He had smoked for 16 years.

Examination

No abnormalities were detected on neurologic examination.

Investigations

Review of magnetic resonance imaging of the brain revealed no abnormalities. An electrocardiogram was normal, and 24-hour Holter monitoring, performed after treatment with indomethacin was started, was also without abnormalities.

Commentary by Dr. David W. Dodick

CPH is an indomethacin-responsive short-lasting trigeminal-autonomic cephalgia. Although trigeminal-autonomic cephalgias share a clinical phenotype—pain in the distribution of the first (ophthalmic) division of the trigeminal nerve and cranial autonomic features—they differ in the frequency and duration of individual attacks and in the differential response to indomethacin. The dramatic response to indomethacin is the clinical hallmark of CPH and reliably distinguishes it from cluster headache.

Indomethacin-responsive headache syndromes represent a unique group of primary headache disorders characterized by a prompt, complete, and often permanent response to indomethacin to the exclusion of other nonsteroidal anti-inflammatory drugs and medications usually effective in treating migraine and cluster headache (Table). They often are confused with cluster headache, as in the case reported here, and are likely more common than previously recognized. Indomethacin-responsive headache syndromes can be divided into several distinct categories. Paroxysmal hemicranias and hemicrania continua invariably respond swiftly and completely to indomethacin, whereas Valsalva-induced and ice-pick headaches may respond in a less consistent fashion.

Paroxysmal hemicranias are characterized by frequent short-lasting unilateral headaches. The female-to-male ratio is approximately 2:1, and the disorder usually begins in adulthood, at a mean age of 34 years. The clinical profiles of CPH and episodic paroxysmal hemicrania are quite similar, the only difference being the presence of pain-free remissions with the latter. The pain is predominantly in the anterior head region (orbital or temporal) and usually lasts between 2 and 45 minutes. The mean duration of an attack is approximately 15 minutes, and the mean frequency of attacks ranges from 5 to 15 per day. This is in contrast to cluster headache, in which less than 6% of headaches last less than 30 minutes and more than 90% of patients have fewer than three attacks per day. About one-third of attacks occur during sleep and often in association with REM sleep.

The pain is strictly unilateral and often very severe. During individual attacks, one or more ipsilateral autonomic symptoms or signs are common. Lacrimation and nasal congestion are the most common accompanying features and are often quite robust. Conjunctival injection and rhinorrhea may occur in one-third of patients. Generalized autonomic dysfunction, including cardiac arrhythmia and syncope, as in the patient presented here, have been described.

Recent evidence from functional neuroimaging studies in patients with cluster headache and SUNCT (short-lasting unilateral neuralgiform headache with conjunctival injection and tearing) syndrome implicates the inferior periventricular hypothalamic gray matter. This region contains the suprachiasmatic nucleus (the human biologic pacemaker), which may well explain the circadian and circannual rhythmic periodicity of these disorders. The descending influence of the hypothalamus on the trigeminal nucleus caudalis and cranial parasympathetic nuclei may explain the clinical phenotype of trigeminal-autonomic cephalgias.

Indomethacin is the treatment of choice for paroxysmal hemicranias and hemicrania continua and has been considered the sine qua non for establishing the diagnosis. The mechanism of its selective effectiveness for certain headache disorders is uncertain. Treatment is usually initiated at a dose of 25 mg three times daily with meals. Treatment response is invariably swift—within 24 hours—once an appropriate dosage is attained. Treatment failure should be considered only if a patient has not had a response to a dosage of 300 mg per day. Maintenance dosages between 25 and 100 mg are usually adequate for maintaining suppression of the headache. For patients who cannot tolerate indomethacin, other medications have been found effective in treating CPH, including acetylsalicylic acid, verapamil, corticosteroids, naproxen, a piroxicam derivative, and acetazolamide.

Table	Indomethacin-Responsive Headache Syndromes

Trigeminal-autonomic cephalgias
 Paroxysmal hemicranias*
  Episodic paroxysmal hemicrania
  Chronic paroxysmal hemicrania
 Hemicrania continua*
 SUNCT (short-lasting unilateral neuralgiform headache with
  conjunctival injection and tearing)
 Cluster headache
  Episodic cluster headache
  Chronic cluster headache
Valsalva-induced headaches
 Benign cough headache
 Benign exertional headache
 Benign sexual headache
Idiopathic stabbing headache (jabs-and-jolts syndrome)

*Indomethacin-responsive trigeminal autonomic cephalgias.

REFERENCE

Boes CJ, Dodick DW. Refining the clinical spectrum of chronic paroxysmal hemicrania: a review of 74 patients. *Headache* 2002;**42**:699-708.

History

A 24-month-old boy presented with no speech, unsteadiness when standing, and a history of seizures since 12 months of age. He was the product of a normal pregnancy, labor, and delivery. He had no speech or syllables, made poor eye contact, and had poor social interactions. He sat at 10 months of age, was able to pull to stand at 17 months, but was unable to walk. He was unsteady in his movements. The seizures occurred when he came out of sleep with jerk-like movements of the arms and then generalized shaking. The seizures were unresponsive to various anticonvulsant agents. He would sleep for only 4 to 6 hours per day and was often awake for much of the night.

Examination

The head circumference was at the 5th percentile and had decreased from the 50th percentile at birth; height and weight were at the 75th percentile. He had poor eye contact, small optic nerves, central hypotonia with peripherally increased tone, decreased but present deep tendon reflexes, down-going plantar responses, and truncal and appendicular ataxia.

Investigations

The blood glucose level was 70 mg/dL (normal, 70-100 mg/dL), and the initial lactate level was 6.1 mmol/L (normal, 0.93-1.65 mmol/L). The lactate measurement was repeated several more times, and the mean level was 4.2 mmol/L; the mean pyruvate level was 0.18 mmol/L (normal, 0.08-0.16 mmol/L). Measurement of serum amino acids showed an increased level of alanine. Ammonia, chromosomes (46 XY), urine organic acids, acylcarnitines, very long chain fatty acids, phytanic acid, and screening tests for Smith-Lemli-Opitz syndrome were all normal. Muscle biopsy results were also normal, including special studies for enzymes of the electron transport chain. Mitochondrial DNA analysis was normal. Electroencephalography showed multifocal spikes and generalized spike-and-wave activity. Findings on magnetic resonance imaging of the head were normal. A skin biopsy specimen failed to show any cytoplasmic inclusions. The electroretinogram was abnormal. An additional laboratory study was performed.

Commentary by Dr. Kenneth J. Mack

If a child presents with hypotonia, myoclonic seizures, and lactic acidosis, a mitochondrial disorder should be strongly considered. However, the results of laboratory tests that often confirm the diagnosis of a mitochondrial disorder, such as muscle biopsy, mitochondrial DNA studies, and magnetic resonance imaging, were normal in this patient. When these tests failed to confirm a diagnosis, additional testing for identifiable causes of autism was undertaken.

Autism is a condition that is identified in infancy and consists of poor social interaction, abnormal language, and unusual behavior, as in the child presented here. Autism can be associated with a long list of causes, but in 94% of patients, the cause is not identifiable. Special chromosome studies are some of the most informative tests in seeking a cause for autism (Figure). As many as 3% of autistic children are fragile X-positive. Fragile X syndrome is a trinucleotide repeat disease caused by expansion of the CGG trinucleotide repeat in the promoter region of the gene for the fragile X mental retardation protein. This X-linked syndrome can affect either boys or girls. This elongated repeat results in methylation of the gene promoter, and methylation results in a transcriptional silencing of the gene. Another potential consideration could have been Rett syndrome, particularly if the child was a girl. Children with Rett syndrome have no speech, difficult-to-control seizures, and hand-wringing behavior, and they also present with apnea. Rett syndrome is also a disorder of methylation caused by the lack of a protein called methyl-CpG-binding protein 2 (MECP2). MECP2 binds to DNA methylated at CpG islands and causes the transcriptional silencing of the downstream genes.

Another consideration in an autistic child is Angelman's syndrome. This was considered likely in the case presented here. A Southern blot test showed an abnormal methylation pattern suggesting an absence of a maternally derived copy of the Prader-Willi/Angelman syndrome region. He was later found to have a microdeletion on chromosome band 15q11.2 by fluorescent in situ hybridization testing, confirming the diagnosis of Angelman's syndrome. Previously, this syndrome was called "the happy puppet syndrome." The clinical spectrum of Angelman's syndrome includes lack of speech, epilepsy, sleep disturbance, slowing of head growth during the first year of life, and a characteristic ataxic, "puppet-like" gait. Recently, lactic acidosis has been reported to be part of the clinical spectrum, particularly in infancy. The molecular defect is the lack of expression of UBE3A, a protein involved in the ubiquitination of other cellular proteins.

In the brain, only the maternally derived allele of this or the *UBE3A* gene is expressed. The paternal allele is silenced by genomic imprinting that occurs early in development. In imprinting, only the allele from one parent is expressed. The other allele is silenced through methylation. Only a small percentage of genes are "imprinted," and although the precise physiologic roles of imprinting are unknown, the process may be important in normal development. Clinical testing involves examining the methylation pattern of the DNA from this genetic region by Southern (DNA) blot. Occasionally, specific DNA probes are used to identify microdeletions in the DNA that result in loss of the maternal allele.

The treatment for the child presented here is supportive. The seizures are difficult to control, but occasionally they respond well to benzodiazepines. Sleep disturbance persists despite behavioral and pharmacologic interventions. Although spoken language never develops, the children can communicate in other ways. Walking usually occurs by 4 or 5 years of age. Genetic counseling is essential to identify other potential carriers.

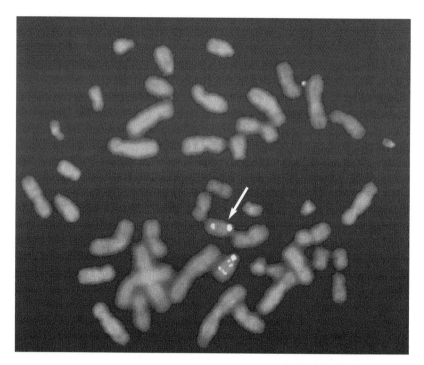

FIGURE. Microdeletion of chromosome 15 in patient with Angelman's syndrome. *Arrow,* The absence of staining of a fluorescent in situ hybridization probe on chromosome 15. This probe covers the genetic region associated with Angelman's syndrome. The absence of staining of this probe on one copy of chromosome 15 implies that the child has a microdeletion of the maternal copy of the gene for Angelman's syndrome (see color insert).

REFERENCE

Clayton-Smith J, Laan L. Angelman syndrome: a review of the clinical and genetic aspects. *J Med Genet* 2003;**40**:87-95.

History

A 79-year-old man had sudden onset of left lower facial weakness, which was followed shortly thereafter by mild weakness of the left arm and leg, moderate dysarthria, and dysphagia. He was transferred to Mayo Clinic after computed tomography (CT) of the head, performed at a local emergency department, showed no evidence of intracranial hemorrhage. He was not given thrombolytic agents. Over a 12-hour period his strength recovered, but he continued to have marked slurring of speech and dysphagia. He had been a smoker in the past and was known to have hyperlipidemia, hypertension, and type 2 diabetes mellitus.

Examination

On neurologic examination, the patient had obvious left lower facial weakness, marked dysarthria, tongue deviation to the left, and mild upper limb ataxia.

Investigations

CT of the head showed evidence of a lacune in the left caudate nucleus. Magnetic resonance angiography demonstrated mild stenosis at the origin of the left internal carotid artery. Transesophageal echocardiography did not show a source of embolism or a patent foramen ovale.

Commentary by Dr. Frank A. Rubino

In this era of high technology, localization in clinical neurology is as important as ever before. First, accurate localization leads to assessment by the least number of appropriate tests. Second, localization leads to the diagnosis of a symptomatic lesion, whereas even proper testing may show other asymptomatic, nonclinically important abnormalities. Third, localization is a very important teaching tool in the education of students of neurology as they gain experience and expertise in the art of obtaining a neurologic history, performing a neurologic examination, and interpreting signs and symptoms.

The condition of the patient presented here quickly improved, but the lingering signs and symptoms that led to localization included left lower facial weakness, dysarthria, dysphagia, and deviation of the tongue to the left. Although the signs and symptoms initially suggest a lesion in the brainstem or even peripheral nervous system, they can well be explained by a cortical lesion in the right frontal operculum (Figure). An acute ischemic infarct in this area suggests a branch occlusion of the right middle cerebral artery from an intrinsic intracranial stenosis or artery-to-artery or cardiogenic embolus. The initial studies did not demonstrate any of these pathophysiologic mechanisms, but later studies demonstrated a possible source in a thickened atheroma of the aorta. The initial weakness and ataxia of the left arm and leg were most likely due to dysfunction of the motor cortex superior to the right frontal operculum and the connection to the cerebellum via the corticopontocerebellar fibers; this may have been on the basis of diaschisis or ischemic "stunning" of the neurons in this area. The old left caudate lacunar infarct and stenosis of the left internal carotid artery were asymptomatic. Indeed, in this case magnetic resonance imaging showed an ischemic infarction in the right anterior operculum.

"Opercula" (plural of "operculum," meaning lid or cover) refers to the region of the cortical mantle and subjacent white matter that surrounds or hides the insular cortex (insula of Reil). It is formed by part of the frontal, temporal, and parietal gyri and, thus, is divided into frontal operculum, temporal operculum, and parietal operculum. A unilateral anterior opercular lesion can cause contralateral facial and lingual weakness along with dysarthria and dysphagia. When the opercular lesions are bilateral, dysphagia tends to last longer and may be permanent, as may be speech difficulties. The anterior opercular syndrome (Foix-Cavany-Marie syndrome) is due to bilateral anterior perisylvian lesions involving the primary motor cortex within the frontal operculum as well as the parietal operculum. This causes facio-pharyngeo-glossomasticatory diplegia with automatic voluntary movement dissociation. The most common causes of this syndrome are multiple strokes, either thrombotic or embolic; other less common causes include tumor, trauma, encephalitis, and congenital anomalies.

A cheiro-oral syndrome has been described with lesions of the parietal operculum, giving rise to contralateral subjective or objective sensory involvement in the peribuccal region and distal part of the upper extremity, mainly the hand and fingers.

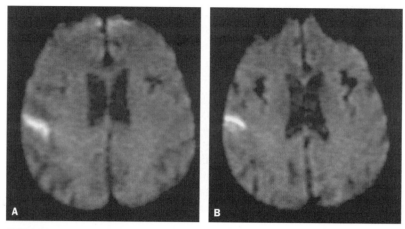

FIGURE. *A* and *B*, Magnetic resonance images demonstrating an infarct in the right anterior operculum.

REFERENCE

Mao CC, Coull BM, Golper LA, *et al.* Anterior operculum syndrome. *Neurology* 1989;**39**:1169-72.

History

A 57-year-old right-handed businessman first noted slowing of his speech 1 year before his death. Within 10 months after the onset of symptoms, he was anarthric but continued to manage his small business and to live alone. Of the five in his sibship, four, including the proband, had impaired language or cognition develop during the sixth decade, and the fifth had benign fasciculations. The patient died 1 year after the onset of symptoms.

Examination

Six months after the onset of symptoms, a severe spastic-flaccid dysarthria developed. He scored 28 of 30 on the Kokmen Test of Mental Status. Although he was anarthric 10 months after onset, he was able to write the answers to questions. Many answers were factually correct but paraphasically misspelled (Figure panel *A*). Twelve months after onset, he had dysphagia and mild weakness of intrinsic hand muscles with few fasciculations. He died later that month.

Investigations

Electromyographic findings were consistent with motor neuron disease. Computed tomography of the brain demonstrated left temporal atrophy (Figure panel *B*).

FIGURE. *A*, Writing sample demonstrating paraphasic spelling of the patient. Patient's written responses to dictation on the left (and the examiner's illegible but linguistically correct scrawl on the right). (From Caselli RJ, Windebank AJ, Petersen RC, *et al. Ann Neurol* 1993;**34**:417-8. By permission of the American Neurological Association.) *B*, Computed tomogram of patient's brain showing left temporal atrophy, correlating with aphasia. (From Caselli RJ, Windebank AJ, Petersen RC, *et al. Ann Neurol* 1993;**33**:200-7. By permission of the American Neurological Association.)

Commentary by Dr. Richard J. Caselli

Dementia within the context of ALS is unusual, but in most cases it is the frontotemporal dementia (FTD) type. This case was even more unusual in that the dementia was a rapidly progressive aphasic variety and was the first example of this type described. Neuropathologic study at autopsy demonstrated widespread cortical gliosis, with loss of neurons and anterior horn cells but relative preservation of the hypoglossal nucleus. The relative sparing of the hypoglossal nucleus suggests that the anarthria was due to upper motor neuron involvement rather than lower motor neuron involvement (which would be more common).

FTD encompasses several distinctive clinical syndromes, including nonfluent aphasia, as in this patient. Pathologically, FTD can be divided roughly into cases that have Pick bodies and other classic features of Pick's disease and cases that lack distinctive histologic features. Within the setting of ALS, FTD typically lacks distinctive histologic features, so the findings in this case were typical. The combination of dementia and ALS in this setting is considered a single disease process rather than dual degenerative diseases simultaneously striking a single patient. Either may be noticed first, but typically dementia occurs early in the course and, in many cases, may precede overt clinical signs of motor neuron disease. FTD differs from Alzheimer's disease in the preponderance of frontal signs such as apathy, abulia, inertia, and, less often, disinhibited behavior. When the disorder is lateralized to the left hemisphere, aphasia may dominate the clinical picture (in most cases), although right hemisphere and bilaterally symmetric cases have been described, too, with a predominantly neuropsychiatric presentation (including Klüver-Bucy syndrome in one case report).

Why some patients have dementia in conjunction with ALS when the majority do not remains unknown, but it has been observed in multiple populations and in familial as well as sporadic cases. The family of this patient included members who had schizophrenia, dementia lacking distinctive histologic features, or a slowly progressive or static dysarthria and one who had benign fasciculations. The relation of phenotypically diverse neurodegenerative syndromes such as dementia, parkinsonism, motor neuron disease, and certain organically based psychiatric syndromes such as schizophrenia and bipolar disorder has been questioned on the basis of kindreds such as this one and others with similar associations, some of which have been found to relate to a mutation of the *tau* gene on chromosome 17. Similarly, the relation between benign fasciculations and motor neuron disease is suspect.

REFERENCE

Caselli RJ, Windebank AJ, Petersen RC, *et al.* Rapidly progressive aphasic dementia and motor neuron disease. *Ann Neurol* 1993;**33**:200-7.

History

A 27-year-old right-handed woman was transferred to the Mayo Clinic Hospital emergency department from a local hospital in generalized status epilepticus. She had no previous history of seizures or epilepsy. In the preceding month, beginning 10 days after the birth of her second child, the patient had experienced four episodes of transient neurologic disturbance that usually lasted 10 to 15 minutes. Typically, the spells began with numbness in her left hand that progressed up her arm, down her left leg, and then to the right side of her body in association with word finding difficulties, severe retro-orbital headaches, nausea, and photophobia. The patient's pregnancy and delivery were without incident except for transient hypothyroidism. She had no history of tobacco, alcohol, or drug use. The family history was unrevealing. The patient's status epilepticus was terminated with propofol and phenytoin. One week after she presented with status epilepticus, she had a recurrent episode of confusion and amnesia that lasted 3 hours.

Examination

After stabilization of the status epilepticus, the only abnormal neurologic finding on examination was difficulty with short-term memory and a mild confusional state in which the patient was alert and oriented but "not herself" according to her husband. The findings on a general neurologic examination were entirely normal. Formal psychometric testing demonstrated short-term memory deficits.

Investigations

The results of computed tomography, magnetic resonance imaging (MRI), and magnetic resonance angiography and venography of the brain and four-vessel angiography were normal. On laboratory testing, a complete blood count, electrolytes, thyroid function, antinuclear antibodies, and the erythrocyte sedimentation rate were normal. The patient had weakly positive antithyroperoxidase antibodies (27 IU/mL; normal, <20 IU/mL). The opening pressure on lumbar puncture was normal, but cerebrospinal fluid (CSF) analysis showed an elevated level of protein (105 mg/dL; normal, 14-48 mg/dL) and glucose (120 mg/dL—serum glucose was 100 mg/dL and normal CSF glucose is 2/3 that of serum glucose). Electroencephalography (EEG) performed several days after status epilepticus showed bifrontal 2- to 3-Hz delta activity in wakefulness and sleep (Figure).

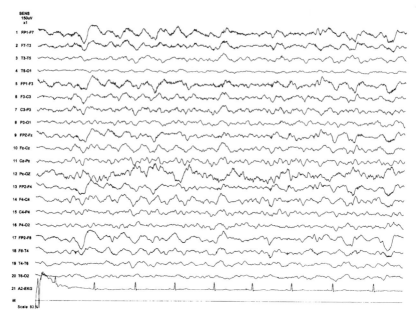

FIGURE. Electroencephalogram showing diffuse slowing and frontal delta activity bilaterally 6 days after successful termination of status epilepticus.

Commentary by Drs. Joseph I. Sirven and Joseph F. Drazkowski

The patient presented with status epilepticus as a manifestation of steroid-responsive encephalopathy associated with autoimmune thyroiditis. This case demonstrates the need to consider an immune-based cause of status epilepticus when no structural or overt lesion is present.

Hashimoto's encephalopathy is a relatively rare disorder (only 50 cases have been reported since 1966), and status epilepticus is an uncommon manifestation of this disorder. Patients with Hashimoto's encephalopathy are typically women in their forties (but it can occur in children and young adults) who present with various episodic neurologic signs and symptoms, including confusion, cognitive disturbance, aphasia, ataxia, focal deficits, myoclonus, tremor, chorea, paralysis, depression, and seizures. The patient had reported four separate episodes of transient neurologic disturbance; however, the findings mimicked those of complicated migraine.

Steroid-responsive encephalopathy is not a diagnosis commonly considered in seizure emergencies. When evaluating causes of status epilepticus, one must rule out infectious, metabolic, vascular, drug-induced, and neoplastic causes. Thyroid function and antibodies (specifically antithyroperoxidase antibodies) should always be examined, even when thyroid function is euthyroid. Antithyroperoxidase antibody titers do not correlate linearly with the severity of the condition. The EEG is abnormal in 89% of patients, with diffuse slowing and frontal slowing being the most commonly reported patterns. The CSF protein level is elevated in 78% of patients. However, MRI findings are commonly normal. Another consideration in this case would have been dural sinus thrombosis. However, in this patient, conventional MRI and magnetic resonance angiography and venography excluded this possibility.

The constellation of signs and symptoms (status epilepticus, episodic neurologic disturbances, abnormal EEG, elevated CSF protein level, and positive antibodies) suggested the diagnosis of Hashimoto's encephalopathy in this patient. This is a treatable disorder. Steroid therapy is effective and is the mainstay of treatment, with the symptoms resolving from 1 day to 4 to 6 weeks after therapy is initiated.

Successful remission occurs in nearly 90% of patients. Indeed, our patient had a response to prednisone therapy within 1 week, which also supported the diagnosis.

REFERENCE

Sawka AM, Fatourechi V, Boeve BF, *et al*. Rarity of encephalopathy associated with autoimmune thyroiditis: a case series from Mayo Clinic from 1950 to 1996. *Thyroid* 2002;**12**:393-8.

History

A 38-year-old African American woman had painful vision loss in the left eye, which was attributed to optic neuritis. She recovered within several weeks after receiving treatment with methylprednisolone intravenously. A baseline magnetic resonance imaging (MRI) study of the brain was normal. Three months later, vomiting and hiccups developed and lasted 4 weeks, but she recovered. No cause was found. One month later, she became quadriparetic over the course of several weeks. She was unable to swallow; respiratory failure developed, and she was intubated. The results of an extensive evaluation were negative. Her condition did not improve with treatment with high-dose methylprednisolone, and she was transferred to Mayo Clinic.

Examination

The patient was alert but ventilator-dependent. She could communicate only by blinking. Her visual acuity appeared to be 20/100 on the left and 20/400 on the right. She had a left gaze paresis but could abduct the right eye. She could protrude her tongue, but the gag reflex was reduced. She had severe flaccid quadriparesis, a left Babinski response, and normal pin sensation.

Investigations

Multiple studies for treatable infections and immune-mediated, metabolic, and genetic disorders were negative. On cerebrospinal fluid analysis, the glucose, protein, and cell count values were normal and no oligoclonal bands were noted. MRI of the head demonstrated a symmetric T_2-signal change involving the upper two cervical spinal cord levels and the majority of the medulla (Figure). The changes extended upward into the right middle cerebellar peduncle, left pons, midbrain, and medial thalamus bilaterally. An additional area of T_2-signal change was seen involving the central cord at T11.

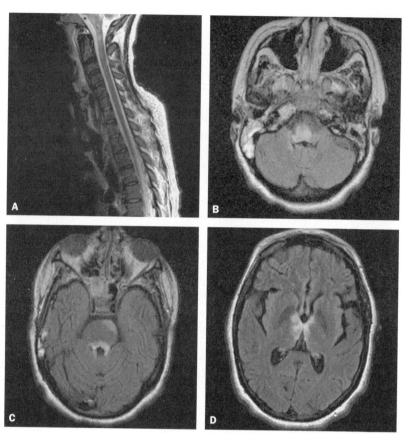

FIGURE. Magnetic resonance images show signal change involving *A*, the upper two cervical cord segments, *B*, most of the medulla, *C*, the pons, and, *D*, the walls of the third ventricle and medial thalami.

Commentary by Dr. Moses Rodriguez

When this patient arrived at Mayo Clinic, she was blind, paraplegic, and in severe respiratory distress. The paraplegia had been present for more than 3 months. Her mother and husband had brought her to Mayo Clinic in hope of a cure. The clinical situation seemed ominous. On MRI, the high cervical-medullary lesion appeared to be demyelinating. The presence of the Fisher one-and-a-half syndrome provided support for this opinion, and the associated optic nerve involvement raised the suspicion specifically of Devic's disease (neuromyelitis optica).

The nosology of Devic's disease is problematic. Previous reports characterized it as a monophasic illness consisting of myelitis and optic neuritis that occurred within months of each other. Recent reports have emphasized that the disease can be similar to multiple sclerosis (MS) and can have clear exacerbations but rare remissions. Initially, the disease was thought to be unique to Asian populations, especially the Japanese. However in the United States, patients of African ancestry are common.

The experience at Mayo Clinic indicates that the disease can be distinguished from MS. Frequently, a longitudinally extensive lesion that is central and may involve more than three spinal segments is seen on MRI of the spinal cord. This type of spinal cord abnormality is unusual in MS. Also, MRI of the head is normal or shows very few lesions consistent with MS. In contrast to MS, patients with Devic's disease frequently have autoantibodies with multiple specificity in their serum. A disease indistinguishable from Devic's disease may develop in patients with classic systemic lupus erythematosus and Sjögren's syndrome. Unlike patients with MS, many patients with Devic's disease have normal cerebrospinal fluid and no oligoclonal bands and may have a pleocytosis consisting of polymorphonuclear cells and occasional eosinophils.

Devic's disease may not respond as well to treatment with interferon-β as MS does. It appears likely that humoral responses may be pathogenic; plasma exchange and azathioprine may be effective, although there are no controlled clinical trials to confirm this opinion.

In my clinical experience, Devic's disease is more frequent and more aggressive in black than in white Americans. We had indirect evidence—based primarily on the prominent vascular changes with immunoglobulin and complement deposition documented in published autopsy studies and on the frequency of associated serum autoantibodies—that the humoral immune response may be pathogenic in this condition. On the basis of the evidence available and the failure of intravenous methylprednisolone therapy to alter the patient's course, plasma exchange was begun without other immune suppression. The results were dramatic. After the second exchange, she was moving the lower extremities, and by the fourth exchange, she was extubated and attempting to walk and her vision was improving. She was discharged to a rehabilitation center on a regimen of interferon-β.

Six months after discharge she was able to walk without assistance and visual acuity had improved so that she could read with corrective lenses. Two years later, however, she had acute worsening of vision and treatment with azathioprine was started, and again her condition seemed to stabilize. While receiving azathioprine and interferon-β, she elected to have breast reduction surgery. This was complicated by a mild exacerbation that responded rapidly to a short course of treatment with intravenous methylprednisolone. In the last several years, her condition has remained relatively stable. She has a mildly ataxic gait and impaired vision in both eyes.

Her striking recovery after months of paraplegia, blindness, and respiratory failure raises important questions about the "window of opportunity" available in the central nervous system for functional recovery even after presumed irreversible deficits. This case demonstrates clearly that recovery from central nervous system injury is possible even after months of deficit and encourages us to continue to work diligently to unravel the basic pathogenesis of neurologic injury and repair even while not knowing the underlying cause of demyelinating diseases of the central nervous system.

REFERENCE

Weinshenker BG, O'Brien PC, Petterson TM, *et al.* A randomized trial of plasma exchange in acute central nervous system inflammatory demyelinating disease. *Ann Neurol* 1999;**46**:878-86.

History

A 43-year-old right-handed woman who had been taking oral contraceptives for 18 months for menorrhagia noted increasing premenstrual headaches for several months. Increasing headaches, nausea, vomiting, loose stools, and sore throat developed. On the day of initial presentation, she noticed slurring of speech and sloppy handwriting, followed 3 hours later by a generalized seizure that started with extension of the right arm. She received treatment with phenytoin at her local hospital. Initially, computed tomography (CT) of the head showed a small cortical hemorrhage, and the cerebrospinal fluid contained numerous erythrocytes. Magnetic resonance imaging (MRI) demonstrated bilateral hemorrhagic cerebral infarctions. Cerebral angiography showed a superior sagittal sinus thrombosis. She received heparin and then warfarin (Coumadin) and rapidly recovered to normal. Over the ensuing 7 months, she continued to have premenstrual headaches, and a repeat imaging study showed the sinus thrombosis. When she presented for a second opinion, she reported that since several days after the initial presentation she had noted a continuous pulse-synchronous unilateral tinnitus that fluctuated with head position.

Examination

A systolic bruit was present over the right mastoid region.

Investigation

A neuroimaging procedure was performed.

Commentary by Dr. Robert D. Brown, Jr.

The positional tinnitus and bruit suggested the diagnosis of DAVF developing as a complication of sagittal sinus thrombosis. The magnetic resonance angiogram and venogram demonstrated very slow flow in the right transverse and sigmoid sinuses. There were enlarged veins in the right jugular foramen. Cerebral angiography demonstrated a large DAVF in the right jugular foramen (Figure). The arterial supply was complex and included feeders from a large anomalous branch of the cervical internal carotid artery and branches from the ascending pharyngeal, posterior auricular, right occipital, and vertebral arteries. Warfarin therapy was discontinued, and a gamma knife procedure was performed. In the subsequent months, the pulsatile tinnitus and bruit disappeared, and she remained well.

Intracranial DAVFs are usually acquired lesions and account for approximately 10% of all intracranial vascular malformations. They form in the wall of a major venous sinus, although smaller veins may also be the nidus of formation. Predisposing factors include venous hypertension, venous outflow obstruction, and venous sinus thrombosis. Often, CT findings are normal, although a contrast study may show some focal enhancement. MRI with magnetic resonance angiography may also be normal, but it can show dilated veins or changes that suggest venous hypertension. The most sensitive study is cerebral arteriography with injection of the vertebral, internal, and, importantly, external carotid arteries.

The clinical presentation is dependent on the site, degree of shunting, and other characteristics of the lesion. Some patients are asymptomatic. Pulsatile tinnitus is a common symptom, particularly with lesions in the transverse and sigmoid sinuses. These symptoms may be minor, although they can become disabling and require either endovascular or surgical management. About 50% of DAVFs have a cranial bruit; overall, however, DAVFs are a relatively uncommon cause of pulsatile tinnitus. Headache, ranging from mild unilateral headaches on the side of the lesion to more severe generalized headaches, may occur. If the superior sagittal sinus is involved, papilledema, vision loss, and pseudotumor may be noted. Cavernous sinus lesions may cause decreased vision, diplopia (due to extraocular muscle dysfunction), chemosis, and proptosis. Focal cranial nerve compression may lead to trigeminal neuralgia or hemifacial spasm. Focal neurologic deficits and seizures are uncommon but may occur with more cortically based lesions. It is important to note that the symptoms can be somewhat nonlocalizing, with intracranial DAVFs occasionally leading to myelopathic symptoms referable to the cervical spinal cord.

One of the outcomes of most concern is intracranial hemorrhage. Hemorrhage is relatively uncommon, occurring at a rate of about 2% per year. The most common site of hemorrhage is intracerebral, followed by subarachnoid and subdural locations. These lesions are complex from an angioarchitectural standpoint, and several arteriographic features have been considered potential predictors of outcome. Predictors of hemorrhage or progressive neurologic deficit include leptomeningeal venous drainage, presence of a venous varix or ectasia, and galenic venous drainage. Petrosal sinus, straight sinus, and tentorial locations may be more likely to be associated with hemorrhage.

Optimal management of a DAVF is based on the site and characteristics of the lesion, the type and severity of symptoms, and the perceived risk of future hemorrhage or progressive deficit. Treatment options include surgical excision, endovascular management, and radiosurgery.

DAVFs can form after venous sinus thrombosis occurs, possibly because the thrombosis and venous obstruction lead to enlargement of the normally tiny arteriovenous shunts in the walls of the venous sinus. If pulsatile tinnitus is reported by a patient following sinus thrombosis, the clinical examination should evaluate for the presence of a cranial bruit. If a bruit is noted in this context, the diagnosis of DAVF should be strongly considered and appropriate imaging studies performed.

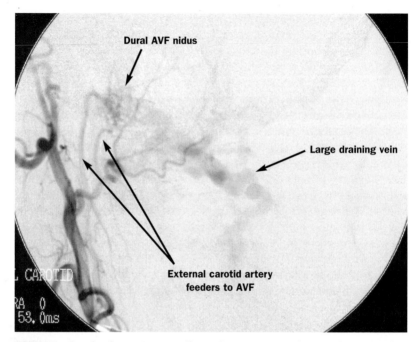

FIGURE. Cerebral arteriogram (lateral view, external carotid injection) showing a dural arteriovenous fistula (AVF) of the right jugular foramen. The fistula had internal and external carotid artery feeders. Drainage was into cervical epidural and suboccipital veins and the inferior jugular vein.

REFERENCE

Awad IA, Little JR, Akarawi WP, *et al.* Intracranial dural arteriovenous malformations: factors predisposing to an aggressive neurological course. *J Neurosurg* 1990;**72**:839-50.

History

A 71-year-old man gave a 4-year history of sleep disturbance. About once a night, his wife would note vocalizations (yelling, profanity) and thrashing of his extremities. Approximately once weekly, he would repeatedly punch the pillow or his wife. He had fallen out of bed on several occasions. He constructed a plywood barrier between his and his wife's side of the bed. If woken, he could recall violent dream content (usually of being attacked) but not the motor activity. He had no history of heavy snoring or restless legs. He felt well rested each morning. He had no symptoms of other neurologic dysfunction.

Examination

The results of neurologic and mental state examinations were normal.

Investigations

Overnight polysomnography with time-synchronized video recording showed markedly increased tone during all episodes of REM sleep (Figure). During one of these episodes, the video recording showed the patient rolling from side to side, shaking his fist in the air, and shouting. No disordered breathing events or periodic limb movements were noted.

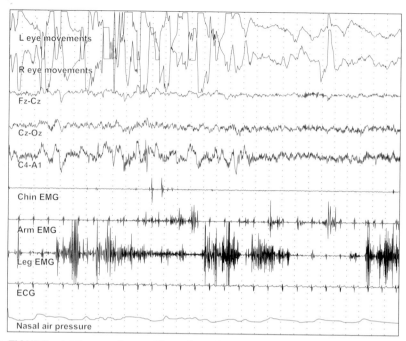

FIGURE. A 30-second recording of a polysomnogram from a patient with REM sleep behavior disorder. The patient is in REM sleep, but electromyographic (EMG) activity is abnormally increased, especially in the leg channel. ECG, electrocardiogram.

Commentary by Dr. Michael H. Silber

The diagnosis of RBD was made, and the patient was treated with clonazepam. With a dose of 0.5 mg before sleep, violent behavior largely ceased. Two years after diagnosis, the patient complained of mild memory problems, and examination showed impaired tests of concentration and learning. He had reduced rapid alternating movements of his tongue and fingers, a positive glabellar tap, bilateral palmomental reflexes, and mild upper limb rigidity. Three years later, a more rapid deterioration of cognitive functions commenced. Neuropsychometric testing confirmed a dementia of subcortical type that progressively worsened over the next 2 years. Dementia with Lewy bodies was diagnosed.

RBD is characterized by dream enactment behavior, including kicking, thrashing, and vocalization. One-third of patients report injuries to themselves, including lacerations, ecchymoses, and occasionally serious trauma such as fractures and subdural hematomas. Two-thirds of bed partners report being assaulted by punches, slaps, kicks, and attempted strangulation. Dream content becomes more violent, most commonly consisting of the patient defending against attack by people or animals. The disorder occurs predominantly in older men, with two large studies reporting mean ages at onset of 52 and 61 years and a male-to-female ratio of 9:1. Diagnosis is confirmed with video-polysomnography, which demonstrates abnormally increased phasic or tonic electromyographic activity during REM sleep, a state normally associated with skeletal muscle atonia.

More than 50% of patients with RBD have an associated neurologic disease. Several lines of evidence suggest that RBD is most commonly associated with neurodegenerative disorders characterized by intracellular inclusion bodies that stain positive for the protein alpha-synuclein. These alpha-synucleinopathies include Lewy body disorders (Parkinson's disease and dementia with Lewy bodies) and multiple system atrophy. RBD occurs in 15% to 33% of patients with Parkinson's disease and in 60% to 90% of those with multiple system atrophy. Prospective and retrospective studies have shown that RBD is often the first manifestation of these disorders, as occurred in the patient presented here. Clinical, neuropsychometric, and pathologic data all indicate that the presence of RBD in a patient with dementia implies that the underlying disease is dementia with Lewy bodies. The dementia is frequently associated with hallucinations and subtle signs of parkinsonism, and psychometric testing shows deficits of attention, perceptual organization, and visual recall. Pathologic examination of brains of these patients demonstrates Lewy bodies, sometimes with additional Alzheimer changes, but there are no reported autopsy cases of pure Alzheimer's disease associated with RBD. Patients with apparent idiopathic RBD are at risk for the development of alpha-synucleinopathies and should be followed closely for evolving symptoms of parkinsonism, cognitive impairment, or dysautonomia.

An essential part of management of RBD is attending to the safety of the bed environment. Furniture should be moved away from the bedside, weapons removed from the bedroom, and consideration given to placing a mattress or large pillows on the floor next to the bed. Clonazepam is effective for the majority of patients but may cause cognitive difficulties, gait unsteadiness, or impotence in older men. Experience with shorter acting benzodiazepines is limited. Case series suggesting success with melatonin have been reported, and sometimes quetiapine may be useful.

REFERENCE

Olson EJ, Boeve BF, Silber MH. Rapid eye movement sleep behaviour disorder: demographic, clinical and laboratory findings in 93 cases. *Brain* 2000;**123**:331-9.

History

A 68-year-old woman presented with a 1-year history of severe, right-sided facial pain localized to the ear, temple, and jaw. The pain was dull and unremitting. On occasion, she experienced sharp fleeting pain localized to the right ear. No aggravating or precipitating factors were known. Initially, she was referred by her internist for a dental opinion. Despite the extraction of several teeth, the pain became increasingly more of a problem, requiring narcotic medications. Subsequently, she was evaluated by a neurologist, who diagnosed trigeminal neuralgia. The results of magnetic resonance imaging of the brain with gadolinium were normal. Sequential trials of therapy with carbamazepine, phenytoin, baclofen, and clonazepam were unsuccessful. Referral for a second neurologic opinion resulted in a diagnosis of atypical facial pain. Therapy with amitriptyline had no effect. The patient had lost 40 lb in the preceding 7 months and complained of early satiety. She had a 40-pack-year smoking history but had not smoked for the past 3 years.

Examination

The findings on neurologic examination were normal. On physical examination, the patient had digital clubbing. A subcutaneous lesion was noted on the right iliac crest.

Investigations

A chest radiograph demonstrated a nodular infiltrate, with volume loss in the right base, affecting primarily the right middle lobe. The erythrocyte sedimentation rate was 36 mm/h (normal range, 0-29 mm/h). Fine-needle aspiration biopsy of the right iliac lesion was performed.

DIAGNOSIS CASE 22
Facial pain secondary to an intrathoracic mass lesion

Commentary by Drs. David J. Capobianco and William P. Cheshire

Facial pain as a presenting symptom of nonmetastatic lung carcinoma was suggested initially by Fay in 1927, who wrote, "I discovered a lesion in the lung... the pain being referred to the face. This may be a coincidence but I suspect not." This association was revived in a case report by Des Prez and Freeman in 1983. A total of 33 cases have been reported.

The clinical features of this underrecognized syndrome have come into sharper focus since the original description by Fay. Of the 30 patients for whom smoking habits were reported, nearly all (91%) were either current or former smokers. The pain, often characterized as a severe aching discomfort, was typically located in or around the ear (91%); other locations included the jaw (48%) and temple (38%). In each case, the pain was ipsilateral to the occult lung lesion. An increased erythrocyte sedimentation rate was noted in 73% (11/15) of patients in whom the test was performed. Nearly 66% of patients for whom data were available met the criteria of the clinical triad of 1) smoking, 2) periauricular pain, and 3) increased erythrocyte sedimentation rate. Additional features that, if present, should raise concern about the possibility of an occult lung lesion include weight loss, new cough or hemoptysis, and digital clubbing.

The mechanism of referral of pain from the chest to the ipsilateral ear or face presumably involves either direct tumor invasion or compression of the vagus nerve (Figure). The vagus is a mixed nerve containing motor, sensory, and parasympathetic components. General visceral afferents project sensory input from the pharynx, larynx, thorax, and abdomen to the nodose ganglion, which then projects to the nucleus solitarius located in the medulla. The jugular ganglion projects general somatic afferents to the nucleus of the trigeminal nerve. The general somatic afferents carry impulses from the skin of the concha of the external ear through the auricular ramus and dura mater of the posterior fossa via the meningeal ramus. Thus, a lung lesion that infiltrates or compresses the vagus nerve may refer pain to the ear through convergence of general visceral afferents and general somatic afferents in the medulla. This dual territory of vagal innervation provides the anatomic substrate for the brain to perceive nociceptive input from the chest as if it were emanating from the ear or meninges.

It behooves clinicians to consider the possibility that facial pain may be related to nonmetastatic lung cancer in every smoker or former smoker with unexplained facial pain or otalgia. All such patients should have chest radiography. If the results are equivocal or negative, computed tomography of the chest should be considered to ensure that an occult lung lesion is not missed. Several cases have been reported recently in which the chest radiograph was normal but chest computed tomography demonstrated an occult lung lesion ipsilateral to the facial pain. Computed tomography was performed in these patients because of a clinical profile of smoking with periauricular pain. In our patient, the chest radiograph was abnormal, but the definitive diagnosis was proven by fine-needle aspiration to be metastatic adenocarcinoma. In general, medical management, including opioids, is largely ineffective in alleviating the pain in such cases. The definitive treatment must be directed at the underlying lung lesion.

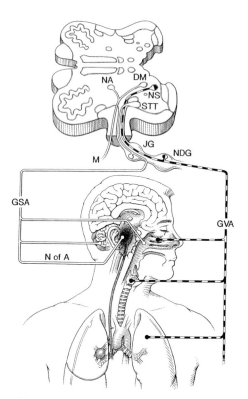

FIGURE. Anatomic connections underlying referred pain from a lung mass to the ipsilateral ear and face. DM, dorsal motor nucleus; GSA, general somatic afferent; GVA, general visceral afferent; JG, jugular ganglion; M, motor fibers; NA, nucleus ambiguus; N of A, nerve of Arnold; NDG, nodose ganglion; NS, nucleus solitarius; STT, spinal trigeminal tract and nucleus. (From Eross EJ, Dodick DW, Swanson JW, *et al. Cephalalgia* 2003;**23**:2-5. By permission of Mayo Foundation.)

REFERENCE

Capobianco DJ. Facial pain as a symptom of nonmetastatic lung cancer. *Headache* 1995;**35**:581-5.

History

A 72-year-old man presented with acute onset of a severe ("thunder-clap") headache. There was no loss of consciousness or evidence of seizures. Computed tomographic (CT) findings showed subarachnoid hemorrhage in the basal cisterns. Placement of a coil into an aneurysm of the anterior communicating artery was successful; however, on post-operative day 5, the patient became paraplegic, drowsy, and mute. Emergency cerebral angiography, with bilateral carotid artery injections, showed proximal vasospasm of the left A-1 and left and right A-2 segments of the anterior cerebral artery. Intra-arterial infusion of papaverine produced some improvement in arterial diameter.

Despite further maximal medical therapy with hemodynamic augmentation with colloids and vasopressors, the patient's condition continued to deteriorate and he died.

Examination

In the emergency department, the patient's Glasgow Coma Score was 15 and examination showed nuchal rigidity. There was no retinal hemorrhage. His condition was World Federation of Neurosurgery grade I. At the time of deterioration, he became abulic and mute and lapsed into sleep when not stimulated. Grasp reflexes and snout reflexes were noted. He had paraparesis, with increased deep tendon reflexes and bilateral Babinski signs.

Investigations

CT of the brain showed diffuse subarachnoid and intraventricular hemorrhage. Cerebral angiography demonstrated an aneurysm of the anterior communicating artery. Diffusion-weighted magnetic resonance imaging at the time of deterioration revealed a hyperintensity in both frontal lobes (Figure). The results of apparent diffusion coefficient mapping were consistent with ischemia.

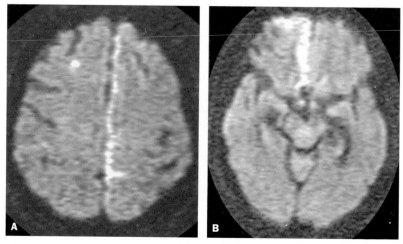

FIGURE. *A* and *B*, Diffusion-weighted magnetic resonance imaging shows hyperintensity in the territory of the anterior communicating artery. This territory corresponded to the area of necrosis found at autopsy.

Commentary by Dr. Eelco F. M. Wijdicks

Cerebral vasospasm and rebleeding are major causes of additional morbidity in patients who survive aneurysmal subarachnoid hemorrhage. There has been a recent emphasis on early surgical or endovascular intervention in the treatment of ruptured cerebral aneurysms. Albeit unproven, there is a perception that this aggressive approach will reduce early rebleeding. If true, cerebral vasospasm will become one of the major remaining causes of deterioration. Early diagnosis of cerebral vasospasm is important and, in certain patients, may lead to effective treatment and prevent permanent infarction.

Initially, management is medical, using hemodynamic augmentation. One way is to use a stepwise approach. This includes infusing large volumes of crystalloids and colloids, vasopressors (to increase mean arterial blood pressure 25% above baseline), and dobutamine (to increase cardiac contractility and performance). The effect of this measure is assessed by cardiac output and systemic vascular resistance data obtained through a pulmonary catheter. Experts believe that early initiation of this protocol will be more effective than initiating it later when symptoms are more severe.

However, a major problem for clinicians is that the initial clinical manifestations of cerebral vasospasm are not distinct. Typically, a decrease in responsiveness predominates. Less common early signs of cerebral vasospasm include such telltale signs as aphasia or hemiparesis. In the case described here, the presentation was even more difficult to grasp. Sudden paraparesis and abulia due to frontal paracentral ischemia are uncommon and, as expected in this circumstance, often puzzling initially. After rupture of an anterior communicating artery aneurysm, paraplegia either is immediately obvious at presentation or occurs with rebleeding and extension of the hemorrhage into the posterior basofrontal areas. In fact, because of the sudden paraparesis, we also suspected that a spinal arteriovenous malformation was causing subarachnoid hemorrhage. More commonly, rupture of an anterior communicating artery aneurysm presents with amnesia and marked behavior abnormality. The clinical presentation may include manic outbursts and compulsive behavior, which may mask the initial onset of headache and delay diagnosis.

Cerebral vasospasm can be implicated in some extraordinary cases, as in the patient considered here. Paraparesis is always associated with abulia, sudden loss of speech, or any other affective disorder, justifying the designation "syndrome." Autopsy of the patient confirmed areas of acute infarction in the frontal cortex characterized by numerous ischemic red neurons, pallor, and minimal vacuolization of underlying parenchyma.

There is a major desire to find better ways to monitor patients at risk for vasospasm. Transcranial Doppler ultrasonography is able to suggest the presence of vasospasm but may not document it in distal arteries. Most importantly, compromised blood supply may not mean neuronal metabolism is compromised and causing ischemia. Affected neurons can increase oxygen extraction, thus countering the threat of ischemia. Newer magnetic resonance modalities for specifically investigating the evolution of ischemia would be welcome. The case described here suggests that, in the appropriate clinical setting, cerebral infarction caused by vasospasm can be confirmed with diffusion-weighted MRI, which may be considered an adjunctive modality in the evaluation of the effects of vasospasm. The presence of ischemic regions should trigger aggressive monitoring of volume status, hemodynamic augmentation, or angiography, followed by angioplasty or intra-arterial infusion of papaverine.

REFERENCE

Greene KA, Marciano FF, Dickman CA, *et al*. Anterior communicating artery aneurysm paraparesis syndrome: clinical manifestations and pathologic correlates. *Neurology* 1995;**45**:45-50.

History

Two years ago, a 47-year-old woman began to notice that she tripped easily but recovered. Nine months before she was evaluated at Mayo Clinic, she developed paresthesias and numbness of both feet and bilateral footdrop after sitting most of the day. Her symptoms improved within hours but did not resolve and seemed to fluctuate considerably daily. At times she noted a fluctuating, more generalized weakness. She also noted intermittent ptosis and chronic headache. For the last 23 years, she was a missionary in East Asia. Six years before the present evaluation, carpal tunnel syndrome was diagnosed after she had spent several days lifting heavy boxes. After a few weeks of treatment with splints, it resolved. Her maternal grandfather developed bilateral footdrop at age 76 years. Electromyography (EMG) had suggested a peripheral neuropathy and bilateral peroneal palsy. Her mother had been told she had carpal tunnel syndrome. Both family members had "high arched feet."

Examination

On examination, the patient had an asymmetric smile, asymmetric weakness of ankle dorsiflexion bilaterally, and mild distal loss of all sensory modalities in all four extremities (legs more than arms). Deep tendon reflexes (except for reduced ankle reflexes), coordination, and gait were normal.

Investigations

The results of extensive investigations for an underlying systemic illness and treatable causes of peripheral neuropathy were normal. Nerve conduction studies showed an absence of median and ulnar sensory responses and low-amplitude sural nerve potentials. Peroneal and tibial motor amplitudes were low. There was marked dispersion and partial conduction block in the left peroneal nerve distal to the fibular head. Focal slowing was seen in the ulnar motor study 4 to 5 cm proximal to the medial epicondyle. Median, ulnar, and peroneal distal latencies were prolonged but not the tibial latency. Conduction velocities were slowed, consistent with a demyelinating polyradiculoneuropathy. Autonomic reflex studies were normal. Fluorescent in situ hybridization (FISH) analysis and sural nerve biopsy were performed. Within a few days after the biopsy, the patient developed severe, burning, distal leg pain that responded slowly and incompletely to treatment with gabapentin.

Commentary by Dr. Jasper R. Daube

The nerve biopsy specimen showed tomaculous neuropathy (Figure), an autosomal dominant, demyelinating neuropathy with liability to pressure palsy (HNPP) that is easily overlooked if the history of recurrent mononeuropathies and a family history of neuropathy are not elicited. FISH analysis confirmed the diagnosis.

The prominent demyelination can lead to a misdiagnosis of the more common Charcot-Marie-Tooth type 1 (CMT1) disease. The genetic defect of the two disorders is related: both have abnormalities of the peripheral myelin protein 22 gene (*PMP22*) on chromosome 17p11.2-12. CMT1 has a duplication of this region, with overexpression of the gene. In contrast, HNPP has a DNA deletion of this segment and underexpression of the gene. An incidence of 16/100,000 population has been reported.

HNPP can occur at any time of life as an acute mononeuropathy, sometimes in patients with a previous history of local compression at a common site of compression, such as the median nerve at the wrist, the ulnar nerve at the elbow, or the peroneal nerve at the knee. However, patients may present with less common mononeuropathies, such as an axillary neuropathy, or with the features of a chronic peripheral neuropathy. Patients often do not relate the new focal deficit to a preceding process, such as the carpal tunnel syndrome in this patient, because the deficits commonly resolve spontaneously over a few weeks. Family members with the disorder may be asymptomatic and unaware of the disorder.

Nerve conduction studies show focal mononeuropathy with conduction block and focal slowing superimposed on the changes of a chronic, diffuse neuropathy. Distal latencies of the median and peroneal nerves are often prolonged out of proportion to more proximal slowing, even without clinical deficits.

Postbiopsy pain occurs in 30% to 40% of patients and usually resolves after a few weeks. The severity and duration of this patient's pain were highly unusual. The neuritic pain following nerve biopsy has not been found to be more common in HNPP than in other neuropathies.

Although the clinical features of some patients are classic, the wide range of presentations of HNPP warrants FISH analysis in atypical disorders with multiple, recurrent mononeuropathies without other causes.

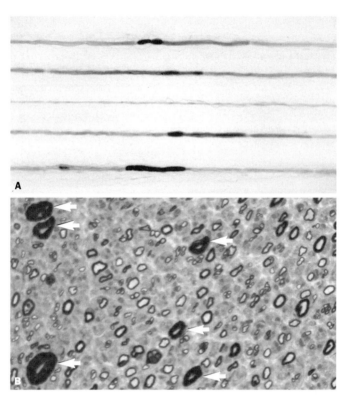

FIGURE. *A*, Teased fibers showing thickened myelin regions (tomaculae). (Original magnification, x12.5.) *B*, Transverse section of sural nerve from the patient. *Arrows*, Large tomaculae, which are regions of reduplication of myelin. The number of myelinated fibers is approximately normal for age. The diameter distribution shows an increased number of intermediate-diameter and excessively large-diameter (tomaculae) fibers (see color insert). (Methylene blue; original magnification, x40.) (The figure is courtesy of Dr. P. J. Dyck and Ms. JaNean Engelstad, Mayo Clinic.)

REFERENCE

Chance PF. Overview of hereditary neuropathy with liability to pressure palsies. *Ann NY Acad Sci* 1999;**883**:14-21.

Case 4

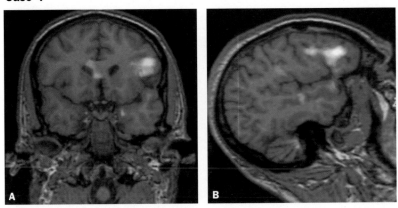

Case 15

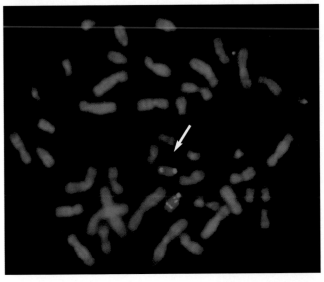

Case 24

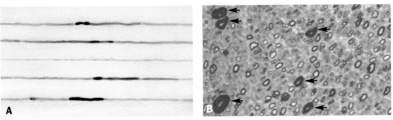

Case 28

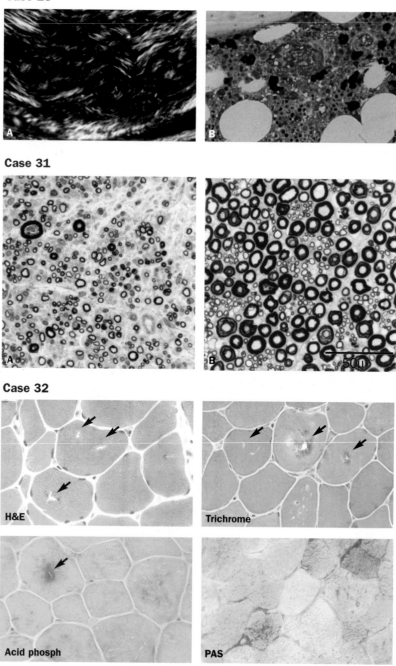

Case 31

Case 32

H&E

Trichrome

Acid phosph

PAS

II Color Insert *Fifty Neurologic Cases From Mayo Clinic*

Case 33

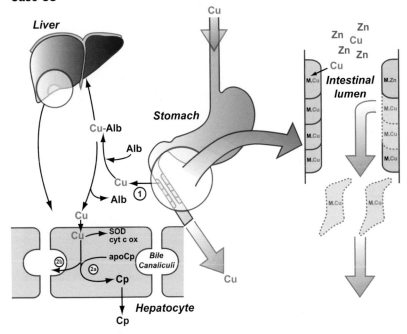

Case 34

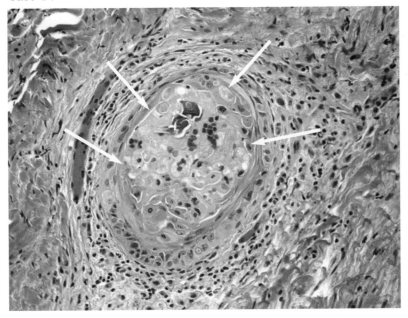

Case 38

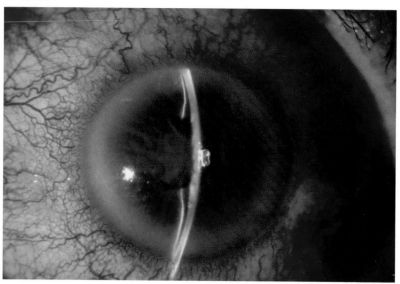

Case 42

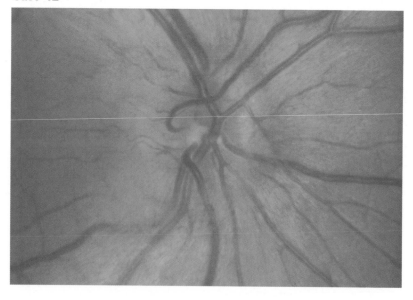

Case 43

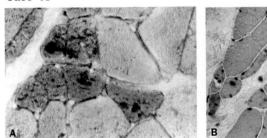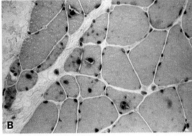

Case 46

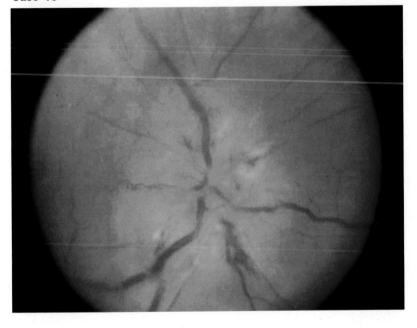

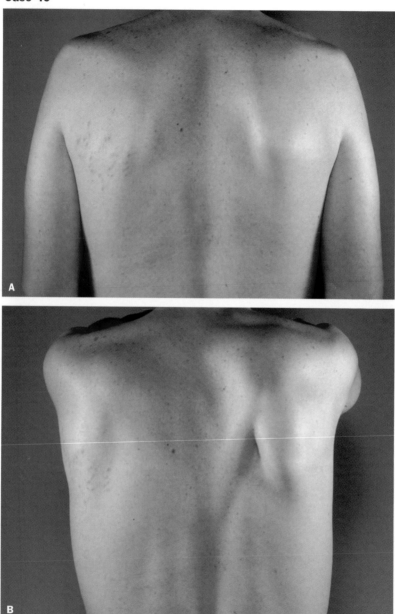

A

B

History

A 30-year-old man presented with a 4-day course of progressive mental status changes and decreased level of consciousness and a 2-day history of dysphagia. He had a history of bronchitis treated with antibiotics 1 month before presentation. His past medical history was otherwise unremarkable. His family history was significant for a transient ischemic attack, due to "occlusive intracranial vascular disease," his mother experienced at age 50. No medical history was known about his father, and his two siblings were healthy.

Examination

On initial examination, the patient was drowsy but aroused to voice. When aroused, he was oriented to self and time. The cranial nerve examination was notable for spastic dysarthria. Motor strength was normal in the upper and lower extremities. Reflexes were normal, with flexor plantar responses. On sensory testing, pain, light touch, and vibratory sensations were intact.

Investigations

Magnetic resonance imaging (MRI) of the head showed multiple bilateral oval lesions, with increased T_2 signal and restricted diffusion in the white matter of both cerebral hemispheres (Figure). Following contrast, enhancement was minimal within the central portion of most of these lesions. Findings on cerebrospinal fluid (CSF) analysis included the following: two white blood cells; protein, 48 mg/dL; and glucose, 71 mg/dL. There was one oligoclonal band, and the IgG index was normal. Other CSF studies were normal. The following studies were performed and were negative or normal: conventional angiography, complete blood count, electrolyte panel, liver function tests, test for human immunodeficiency virus, rheumatologic screen, erythrocyte sedimentation rate, thrombotic coagulation panel, and drug screen. His total cholesterol was 274 mg/dL. A diagnostic study was performed.

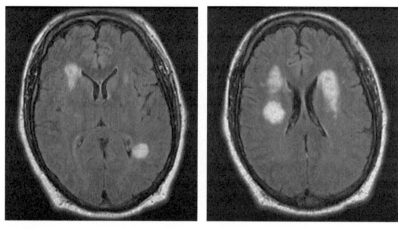

FIGURE. Magnetic resonance imaging of the head shows increased FLAIR signal in the deep white matter.

DIAGNOSIS CASE 25
**Cerebral autosomal dominant arteriopathy with subcortical
infarcts and leukoencephalopathy (CADASIL)**

Commentary by Dr. Kelly D. Flemming

The patient initially received treatment with corticosteroids for presumed acute disseminated encephalomyelitis (ADEM). After treatment was initiated, skin biopsy results became available. Electron microscopy showed thickening of the basal lamina from deposits of granular osmophilic material (GOM), consistent with CADASIL.

CADASIL is an inherited condition characterized by migraine, recurrent subcortical strokes, and dementia. The disease leads progressively to a subcortical dementia characterized by frontal lobe signs and memory loss. In addition, pseudobulbar palsy, gait disturbance, pyramidal signs, and urinary incontinence may be present. MRI studies generally show increased T_2-signal changes in the deep white matter (especially the periventricular area) and basal ganglia. It has been suggested that another useful diagnostic marker is involvement of the anterior temporal pole seen on MRI. Pathologically, there is evidence of widespread myelin pallor of the white matter and multiple small infarcts in the white matter and basal ganglia, which are generally symmetric. The vessels of the white matter and meninges are thickened, and the media of the vessels is characterized by a smudgy granular material and the loss of smooth muscle cell nuclei. GOM is visible with electron microscopy and is of uncertain significance.

CADASIL results from mutations in the *Notch3* gene on chromosome 19. This gene codes for a transmembrane protein involved in intercellular signaling essential for control of cell fate during development.

Although patients with CADASIL typically present with the symptoms noted above, they may present also with encephalopathy and coma. The patient described here presented with a reduced level of consciousness and focal neurologic signs (dysphagia). Schon et al. reported six patients with CADASIL who presented with encephalopathy or coma. All six had confusion at presentation, four had headache at onset, four had fever, and four had seizures. Additional case reports have noted similar presentations with self-limited episodes. In these patients, CADASIL often was misdiagnosed as acute encephalitis or ADEM (or both), as it was in the patient described here.

Clinical features suggested to help differentiate CADASIL from other entities include the family history, a personal or family history of migraine headaches, and topography of MRI findings. White matter changes involving the anterior temporal pole and external capsule are thought to help distinguish between CADASIL and leukoariosis radiographically. One study has suggested that involvement of the anterior temporal lobe has a sensitivity of 89% and specificity of 86% for the diagnosis of CADASIL. In the patient described here, the lack of an extensive family history, the absence of migraine headaches, and no radiographic evidence of involvement of the anterior temporal lobe made a clinical diagnosis of CADASIL difficult.

Other investigations that may help establish the diagnosis of CADASIL include skin biopsy and genetic testing. On electron microscopy, GOM is characteristic of CADASIL. Skin biopsy findings are 100% specific but approximately only 45% sensitive for making the diagnosis. To increase the sensitivity of skin biopsy, investigators are immunostaining arterioles with a Notch3 monoclonal antibody. Although this is not widely available, it may be useful.

Genetic testing can be time-consuming and expensive because of the size of the *Notch3* gene, which contains 33 exons encoding for a protein of 2,321 amino acid residues. The mutations in CADASIL have been associated with the first 23 exons, but screening for all 23 exons can be difficult. Because nearly 70% of all mutations occur at exon 4, it has been recommended that screening for CADASIL begin with this exon and proceed to exons 3, 5, and 6 when indicated.

Although patients with CADASIL typically present with migraine, focal deficits, or progressive dementia, skin biopsy and genetic testing should be considered to evaluate for CADASIL in patients with acute encephalopathy and white matter changes.

REFERENCE

Schon F, Martin RJ, Prevett M, *et al*. "CADASIL coma": an underdiagnosed acute encephalopathy. *J Neurol Neurosurg Psychiatry* 2003;**74**:249-52.

History

At age 51 years, a woman began to notice that she had trouble pronouncing "puh" and "buh" sounds. She experienced progressive fatigue and developed tingling in several fingers, first in the left hand and then in the right hand. Eyelid closure was found to be weak. She could not whistle, and her hands were weak. Later she noted that she was not able to purse her lips to apply lipstick and her trunk, arms, and face were numb. Progressive numbness and weakness of her hands and face and intermittent dysarthria and dysphagia developed. Bladder and bowel function and gait were spared. The results of extensive studies, including myelography and bone marrow biopsy, were normal. She did not have a response to corticosteroid therapy. At age 62, she noted that her left nostril felt "closed," her throat seemed irritated, and her right leg felt that it might give way. Her hands seemed cold and heavy; episodically, these sensations were interrupted by brief jabbing pains. Her eyes were not excessively dry. Her past medical, social, and family histories were unremarkable.

Examination

The corneas were cloudy. There was facial diplegia and moderate bilateral distal hand weakness and wasting. The motor examination of the legs was normal. Superficial pain sensation was markedly reduced above the waist, including the face and scalp. Tongue sensation was normal. Vibration sense and joint position sense were normal in the hands, but vibration sense was reduced from the feet to the level of the ankles. Deep tendon reflexes, coordination, gait, and station were normal.

Investigations

The results of extensive biochemical and hematologic studies were normal. The results of a rectal biopsy to examine for amyloid were inconclusive. Motor conduction studies demonstrated no response from the median and ulnar nerves, but responses were normal from the musculocutaneous, peroneal, and posterior tibial nerves. Sensory conduction was decreased in the median nerve but normal in the sural nerve. On needle examination, neurogenic changes were found in left arm muscles. Esophageal motility was normal. An ophthalmologist diagnosed exposure keratitis. A sural nerve biopsy specimen demonstrated a decrease in the number of myelinated fibers, with evidence of segmental remyelination. A diagnostic blood test and biopsy were performed.

Commentary by Dr. Peter J. Dyck

The patient has late-onset Tangier disease, a rare, autosomal recessively inherited, multisystem disorder, presenting neurologically as a primary axonal degeneration of unmyelinated (dorsal root and sympathetic) fibers, small (Aσ) and large (Aαβ) sensory fibers, and motor fibers, especially of the bulbar, cervical, and thoracic levels (Figure). Tangier disease was first described in 1960 in children from Tangier Island (Virginia) in the Chesapeake Bay. Their removed tonsils contained macrophages with excessive cholesterol esters. The increased cholesterol deposition was linked to extremely low levels of serum high-density lipoprotein (HDL) cholesterol. The molecular genetic defect that explains the clinical disorder is due to mutations in both alleles encoding a lipid transporter called "ABCA1." A related lipid disorder, familial HDL deficiency (also called "familial hypoalph-alipoproteinemia" [FHA]), occurs in persons who have one normal and one mutant allele encoding ABCA1.

Fewer than 100 cases of Tangier disease have been reported. The patients have a sixfold increased risk of developing coronary artery disease in middle or old age.

Neuropathy associated with Tangier disease has been classified into three subtypes: 1) an asymmetric relapsing-remitting mononeuropathy; 2) a symmetric, slowly progressive polyneuropathy of the lower limbs, with preferential involvement of small fibers; and 3) a disorder, usually of middle or late life, predominantly affecting the face, neck, and thorax, with facial diplegia, hand weakness and atrophy, and dissociated sensation (greater loss of pain and temperature sensation than of mechanosensation). Sudomotor function is also abnormal in the affected region. With time, the sensory loss becomes increasingly pan modality and extends to other regions of the body. This "pseudosyrinx" phenotype is rare and perhaps most severe. The case reported here is an example of the third subtype of Tangier disease.

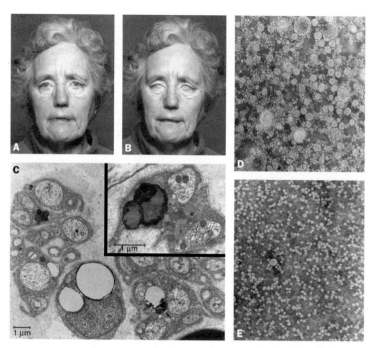

FIGURE. Tangier disease. *A* and *B*, Marked facial weakness is noted when the patient attempts to smile (*A*) and close her eyes (*B*). *C*, Note membrane-bound lipid droplets in Schwann cells, possibly at former sites of unmyelinated fibers. The inset shows lipofusion in a small Remak bundle. *D*, Negatively stained lipoprotein particles. Compare them with particles from a control subject (*E*). (*A-C* from Dyck PJ, Ellefson RD, Yao JK, *et al. J Neuropathol Exp Neurol* 1978;**37**:119-37. *D* and *E* from Yao JK, Herbert PN, Fredrickson DS, *et al. J Neuropathol Exp Neurol* 1978;**37**:138-54. By permission of the American Association of Neuropathologists.)

REFERENCE

Dyck PJ, Ellefson RD, Yao JK, *et al.* Adult-onset of Tangier disease: 1. Morphometric and pathologic studies suggesting delayed degradation of neutral lipids after fiber degeneration. *J Neuropathol Exp Neurol* 1978;**37**:119-37.

History

Over several weeks, a 35-year-old man developed progressive neurologic symptoms. These included supine occipital headache with nausea and vomiting, ataxia of gait such that he was unable to walk unaided, vertical diplopia, and hoarseness of voice. He lost 30 lb. He had a long-standing history of alcohol and nicotine dependence and a 10-year history of hypertension. His mother had had an operation for a brain tumor. Studies performed before his evaluation at Mayo Clinic included magnetic resonance imaging (MRI), cerebrospinal fluid analysis (normal results), and four-vessel and aortic arch cerebral angiography (normal findings).

Examination

On examination, his eye movements were ataxic, with direction-changing, asymmetric horizontal nystagmus. The palate and tongue deviated to the left, and his voice was hoarse. Examination also demonstrated right arm dysmetria, left-sided hyperreflexia, flexor plantar responses, and severe gait ataxia (the patient was unable to stand unassisted). Findings on the sensory examination were normal.

Investigations

MRI of the brain demonstrated increased T_2 signal and expansion of the medulla bilaterally, greater on the right, with nodular patchy enhancement following the administration of a contrast agent (Figure 1).

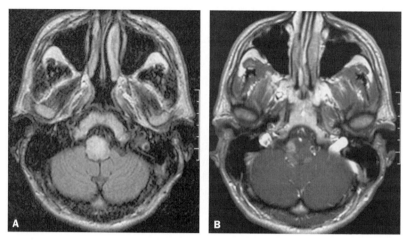

FIGURE 1. *A* and *B,* Initial MRI study showing increased T$_2$ signal and expansion in the medulla with patchy enhancement following the administration of gadolinium.

Commentary by Dr. Brian A. Crum

The diagnosis was suggested in part by finding, on the cervical MRI study, dilated vessels within the upper cervical spinal canal extending from the level of the brainstem to C5 (Figure 2). Selective cerebral angiography identified, at the level of the left pontomedullary junction, a small high-flow DAVF supplied by the left vertebral artery, with left meningeal and left anterior inferior and posterior inferior cerebellar artery trunk feeder vessels and a small contribution through collateral vessels from the left external carotid artery.

At surgery, an arterialized vein that extended from the dura mater to the brainstem at the pontomedullary junction was identified. This vein, as well as the identified feeding vessels, were coagulated and divided. Postoperatively, the patient was independent in ambulation and did not experience nausea but continued to have mild ataxia and a deviated palate. One week postoperatively, angiography was repeated and the findings were normal. Three months later, an MRI study of the brain showed near-complete resolution of the abnormal signal in the brainstem and complete resolution of the abnormal vascular signals in the cervical spine. At this time, the patient's gait and appendicular ataxia had improved but the palate still deviated to the left.

DAVFs are shunts from a dural arterial supply to a dural venous supply. The presentations vary; DAVFs can affect all levels of the central nervous system as well as the cranial nerves and nerve roots. Drainage of DAVFs may be into venous sinuses (e.g., cavernous and sigmoid sinuses) or into cerebral or perimedullary veins. Although DAVFs usually arise spontaneously, they may result from a congenital anomaly. Proper hemodynamic circumstances are required for their delayed development. In some instances, either a sinus thrombosis or venous sinus hypertension may lead to their formation.

Although intracerebral arteriovenous malformations lead to a "steal" phenomenon because of their high flow rates, a DAVF has a relatively slow flow rate and the steal phenomenon is thought not to be sufficient to lead to symptoms referable to the central nervous system. However, cranial neuropathies, which occasionally are related to DAVFs, may be caused by a "steal" from meningeal dural arteries. Within the brain, excessive blood flow due to a DAVF may lead to the classic combination of pulsatile tinnitus, headache, and cranial bruit.

Also, dural venous lakes can produce a mass effect. Venous sinus hypertension may develop, which can lead in turn to impaired cerebrospinal fluid absorption, hydrocephalus, and papilledema. Venous sinus thrombosis can also occur, especially in a cavernous sinus DAVF. Hemorrhage, including subarachnoid hemorrhage, can be a serious complication.

The main detrimental effect of DAVF is likely from venous hypertension and resultant ischemia. Passive congestion occurs from retrograde, increased venous pressure toward the venous drainage routes of the normal brain and spinal cord. Because intramedullary veins lack valves, they are affected even more directly by increased pressure in perimedullary veins.

Cases of intracranial DAVF with perimedullary drainage are rare, and a review in 1999 documented 37 reported cases. We have examined a few cases at Mayo Clinic. Either myelopathy or hemorrhage is universally present, and sphincter disturbances are common. Bulbar signs, ataxia, and autonomic dysfunction are found less frequently. MRI shows T_2 hyperintensity in the rostral spinal cord and medulla, although enhancement and the lack of spinal cord T_2-signal changes, as in our case, are unusual.

A constant feature is that the site of T_2-signal change does not necessarily indicate the site of the DAVF, a useful point to remember because full-neuraxis imaging is warranted if the diagnosis of DAVF is being considered. In our patient, extended neuroimaging was crucial because before the results of cervical spine MRI were known, biopsy of the medulla was being considered to evaluate the presumptive diagnosis of neoplasm.

The goal of treatment of this type of DAVF is to disconnect the draining vein, thereby eliminating the fistula. Both embolization and direct surgical disconnection have been advocated. Success rates, even at experienced centers, may be slightly lower with embolization than surgery, although both are successful in nearly 70% to 95% of cases. A direct surgical approach has low rates of failure or morbidity or mortality and, thus, is the treatment of choice at our institution.

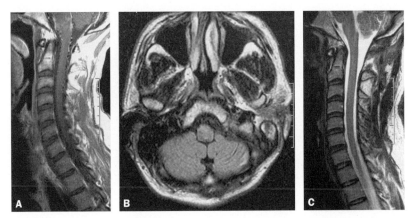

FIGURE 2. *A*, Sagittal MRI of cervical spine showing enhancing serpiginous vessels on the surface of the spinal cord. *B* and *C*, Postoperative MRI showing resolution of the T_2 hyperintensity in the medulla (*B*) and of the abnormal vascular signals in the cervical spine (*C*).

REFERENCE

Ricolfi E, Manelfe C, Meder JF, *et al*. Intracranial dural arteriovenous fistulae with perimedullary venous drainage: anatomical, clinical and therapeutic considerations. *Neuroradiology* 1999;**41**:803-12.

History

A 52-year-old man who had diabetes mellitus presented with insidious onset of orthostatic hypotension and syncope of several years' duration. Midodrine hydrochloride and compressive stockings were minimally helpful. He complained of ice-pick jabbing foot pain, paresthesias, and numbness in his feet. He had suffered painless burn injuries. Recently, he developed similar sensations in his hands and nocturnal diarrhea, leading him to wear diapers. He was impotent and had recently lost 40 lb. He had an 8-year history of diabetes mellitus requiring insulin therapy, and he was a smoker. He had no visual symptoms or known kidney disease. One sister had recently developed proteinuria.

Examination

He was cachectic. His blood pressure while sitting was 120/100 mm Hg (pulse, 65 beats/min) and while standing, 90/80 mm Hg (pulse, 70 beats/min). He had no retinopathy. Examination showed mild distal weakness in the hands and feet, with marked loss of proprioception and light touch distally, especially in the legs. The Romberg test was positive.

Investigations

Glycosylated hemoglobin and serum creatinine values were normal. No proteinuria was detected at the time of presentation. The findings of nerve conduction and needle electromyographic studies were consistent with a sensory-greater-than-motor, length-dependent, axonal-predominant neuropathy, as evident by predominant loss of sensory nerve action potentials and minimal distal neurogenic potentials on needle examination. Autonomic testing showed severe cardiovagal and cardiovascular adrenergic impairment with length-dependent, postganglionic sympathetic sudomotor involvement. Thermoregulatory sweat studies demonstrated anhidrosis below the knee. Gastric emptying was delayed. A fat aspirate was negative for amyloid, and serum and urine immunofixation were negative for monoclonal proteins. Computed tomography of the chest showed no abnormality, and paraneoplastic antibody studies, including ganglionic nicotinic-cholinergic antibody, which may be associated with primary lung carcinoma (small cell) and dysautonomia, were normal. Additional diagnostic studies were performed.

Commentary by Dr. Christopher J. Klein

A sural nerve biopsy specimen demonstrated decreased fiber density, with acellular thickened microvessels that were apple-green birefringent under polarized light when stained with Congo red (Figure). A bone marrow biopsy demonstrated a λ B-cell dyscrasia and amyloid fibril staining specific for λ amyloid. DNA sequencing of the entire expressed region of transthyretin gene (*TTR*) was normal.

The causes of autonomic polyneuropathy are diverse and can be divided broadly into inherited and acquired forms. Because of the patient's insidious course, with prominent gastrointestinal symptoms, weight loss, and superimposed painful length-dependent polyneuropathy, systemic amyloidosis was the major consideration. The negative amyloid fat aspirate did not dissuade us from considering this diagnosis. Paraneoplastic autonomic neuropathies may also be associated with weight loss, but they commonly occur subacutely and are typically without length-dependent features. The extent of the patient's sensory and motor involvement would also make idiopathic autonomic failure or pure autonomic failure an unlikely diagnosis. Diabetes may present with this constellation of symptoms, signs, and temporal course but would be unusual without retinopathy, nephropathy, or abnormal glycosylated hemoglobin values.

Although many forms of systemic amyloidosis have been described, only two are readily recognized to produce autonomic neuropathy, namely, AL amyloidosis (also referred to as primary or light chain amyloidosis, associated with monoclonal immunoglobulins) and inherited transthyretin amyloidosis. The information that his sister was alleged to have proteinuria raised the possibility of the familial form. Also, the absence of immunoglobulins in his urine and serum made the inherited form seem more likely because immunoglobulins are identified in approximately 85% to 90% of patients with AL amyloidosis.

The diagnostic dilemma centered on the specific form of amyloidosis identified. Only after the bone marrow had been examined was a λ B-cell dyscrasia identified. Immunophenotyping of the bone marrow amyloid fibrils clarified the diagnosis of AL amyloidosis, λ type. Although the patient was relatively young, it is important to note that identification of a paraprotein in older patients may be misleading because it is sometimes observed in older healthy persons. One should not assume that an identified paraprotein is the cause of amyloidosis. Conversely, as illustrated in this case, the absence of paraproteins cannot exclude AL amyloidosis. Immunophenotyping the amyloid fibril is important in identifying the specific origin of an amyloid protein. However, phenotyping may be difficult technically in some patients. Increasingly, genetic testing is becoming important in identifying the hereditary forms of amyloidosis. We sequenced our patient's entire open reading frame for the transthyretin gene. Currently available commercial testing is inadequate to exclude all disease-causing mutations. This was done in part because of the sister's proteinuria, which may be the first feature of transthyretin amyloidosis. No mutation was found.

A recent study has attempted to determine how many cases of inherited amyloidosis were initially mislabeled as AL amyloidosis. The authors sequenced the DNA of 350 patients in whom AL amyloidosis had been diagnosed and identified 13 with point mutations in the transthyretin gene. None of these 13 had undergone original confirmatory immunophenotyping of the amyloid protein and most had paraproteins. The absence of a family history should not exclude consideration of the diagnosis of inherited amyloidosis because clinical ascertainment in family members and de novo mutations may obscure the diagnosis. Identifying the specific form of amyloidosis is important to patients and their families. Because the abnormal protein is synthesized in part in the liver, patients with the transthyretin form may receive benefit from a liver transplant. In general, patients with the transthyretin form tend to fare better than those given chemotherapy for AL amyloidosis. Typically, life expectancy is less than 5 years from the time of diagnosis of orthostatic hypotension in AL amyloidosis. Despite chemotherapy, the patient died within 3 years after he first had symptoms of orthostatic hypotension.

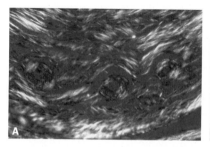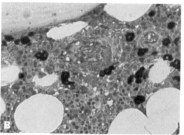

FIGURE. *A,* Sural nerve biopsy specimen stained with Congo red and viewed with a polarized light filter. Note the prominent apple-green birefringence of endoneurial microvessels. *B,* Bone marrow biopsy specimen stained with antiserum for λ amyloid fibrils demonstrates a prominent B-cell λ plasma-cell population. Microvessel amyloid staining was not seen with comparable stains for κ and transthyretin (see color insert).

REFERENCE

Lachmann HJ, Booth DR, Booth SE, *et al.* Misdiagnosis of hereditary amyloidosis as AL (primary) amyloidosis. *N Engl J Med* 2002;**346:**1786-91.

History

A 10-year-old girl presented with a 5-year history of daily headaches. One to three times daily she had a sudden severe headache, photophobia, nausea, and vomiting and needed to lie down. One year ago, she was thought to have papilledema and enlarged blind spots. Repeated lumbar punctures demonstrated an increase in cerebrospinal fluid (CSF) pressure, with moderate pleocytosis (60-200 cells); repeated culture studies were negative. After each lumbar puncture, the headaches improved for 4 to 12 weeks. Acetazolamide was prescribed along with a course of corticosteroid therapy but was without benefit. She was a slow learner and had been placed on a special education track. Since infancy, she has had recurrent erythema multiforme and eczema. She also has a 3-year history of arthralgia and arthritis with effusions (one elbow and both knees), typically lasting 1 or 2 days and accompanied by fever, redness of the eyes, and occasionally erythema multiforme, and a 2-year history of bilateral sensorineural hearing loss requiring hearing aids.

Examination

Her speech and social skills were thought to be appropriate for a 6-year-old child. There was chronic papilledema without loss of visual acuity or optic atrophy. Visual fields were normal. She had bilateral sensorineural hearing loss.

Investigations

The following was found on CSF analysis: opening pressure, 44 cm H_2O; 129 leukocytes (57% segmented cells, 7% lymphocytes, 27% monocytes, and 9% eosinophils); glucose, normal; protein, mildly elevated; and Gram stain, culture studies (bacterial, viral, mycobacterial, brucellar), and the polymerase chain reaction for cytomegalovirus, Epstein-Barr virus, herpes simplex virus, and varicella-zoster virus were negative. No abnormalities were detected with mitochondrial DNA mutation analysis. A diagnostic study was performed.

Commentary by Dr. Nancy L. Kuntz

The patient was referred for evaluation of recurrent aseptic meningitis. Careful review of her clinical course demonstrated that she had chronic meningitis associated with polymorphonuclear cell infiltration, no identifiable organism on repeated culture studies and immunocytochemistry of the CSF, and multisystem involvement. Repeated bacterial, fungal, and viral cultures of the CSF and polymerase chain reaction of the CSF for multiple organisms, including cytomegalovirus, Epstein-Barr virus, herpes simplex virus, varicella-zoster virus, and enterovirus, had not been revealing. Multisystem involvement included chronic intermittent rashes, which appeared initially in the newborn nursery; sensorineural deafness noted at age 6 years; arthralgias, with a history of arthritis in her hands at age 7 years; and global developmental delays.

Clinical suspicion led to testing of the *CIAS1* gene, which codes for cryopyrin. The results confirmed the diagnosis of cryopyrin-associated disease. In this case, a V262A mutation was detected in the *CIAS1* (cryopyrin) gene.

Cryopyrin-associated disease represents a clinical spectrum of autoinflammatory disorders not associated with autoantibodies or antigen-specific T cells (Table). Within the past few years, several clinical disorders have been found to be associated with *CIAS1* mutations, from familial cold autoinflammatory syndrome at the mild end of the clinical spectrum to Muckle-Wells syndrome to chronic infantile neurologic cutaneous articular syndrome (CINCA) at the severe end of the spectrum. CINCA has also been termed "neonatal-onset multisystem inflammmatory disease" (NOMID).

CINCA, or NOMID, is characterized by the clinical triad of neonatal onset of an intermittent urticaria-type rash, arthropathy caused by cartilaginous abnormalities leading to bony overgrowth, and neurologic involvement. The urticaria-type rash nearly always appears within the first few months of life, frequently within the first few hours. Classically, the arthropathy occurs in the knees but can involve multiple other joints. The neurologic symptoms are thought to result from chronic aseptic meningitis, with subsequent high-frequency hearing loss, chronic papilledema, and eventual cerebral atrophy with hydrocephalus ex vacuo and developmental delay.

Within the past several years, the majority of patients with cryopyrin-associated disease have been shown to have a missense mutation of the *CIAS1* gene. Cryopyrin belongs to a family of proteins involved in the regulation of inflammation, the processing of cytokines, and apoptosis. Other clinical disorders etiologically linked to mutations in this family of proteins include familial Mediterranean fever (pyrin protein mutations) and tumor necrosis factor receptor-associated periodic syndrome. The *CIAS1* gene is expressed primarily in polymorphonuclear cells and chondrocytes, which explains the clinical abnormalities in the regulation of inflammation and in the formation of cartilage. Cryopyrin-associated diseases have demonstrated autosomal dominant inheritance, but a majority of children with NOMID/CINCA appear to have de novo mutations.

In our patient, a complete bidirectional sequence analysis of exon 3 of the *CIAS1* gene was performed by Gene DX DNA Diagnostic Services. A heterozygous change identified at position 262 was expected to lead to substitution of alanine for the normal valine at that position in the cryopyrin protein (V262A). This particular mutation has not been described previously.

NOMID/CINCA is a chronic inflammatory disorder. Progressive symptoms include deafness, visual impairment caused by an ocular inflammatory disorder, progressive neurologic impairment due to chronic meningitis, and deforming arthropathy. The reported causes of death have included amyloidosis, vasculitis, and infection. Treatment has been difficult because nonsteroidal anti-inflammatory medications and corticosteroids have not been effective for most patients. In our patient, a gradual decrease in the CSF neutrophil count was noted during an interval of treatment with oral corticosteroids; however, chronic meningitis and symptomatic increased intracranial pressure persisted. After the diagnosis of NOMID/CINCA was made, a trial of oral colchicine was initiated.

Table Comparison of Features of Syndromes of Cryopyrin
Mutations

	FCAS	MWS	NOMID
Skin	Cold urticaria	Urticaria	Neonatal-onset urticaria
CNS	---	SN deafness	Chronic aseptic meningitis, papilledema, SN deafness
Joints	Arthralgia	Synovitis	Premature epiphyseal ossification

CNS, central nervous system; FCAS, familial cold autoinflammatory
syndrome; MWS, Muckle-Wells syndrome; NOMID, neonatal-onset
multisystem inflammatory disease; SN, sensorineural.

REFERENCE

Hull KM, Shoham N, Chae JJ, *et al.* The expanding spectrum of systemic autoinflammatory disorders and their rheumatic manifestations. *Curr Opin Rheumatol* 2003;**15**:61-9.

History

A 38-year-old man had subacute onset of headache and behavior change. Initially, he complained of headache, word-finding difficulty, and oscillopsia. He became increasingly inattentive and confused; demonstrated repetitive, nonproductive behavior; and had vertigo, gait disturbance, and vomiting. Within 1 month after onset, he showed poor judgment, became more withdrawn, and complained of left-sided hearing loss. His past personal and family medical histories were unremarkable.

Examination

The mental status examination demonstrated problems involving multiple tasks, including orientation, attention, calculations, abstraction, and learning. He was abulic. Retinal arteriolar occlusions were noted in the right eye. Hearing was reduced on the left. Gait was ataxic.

Investigations

Electroencephalography demonstrated generalized slowing. Fluorescein angiography showed right inferior temporal artery occlusion, with localized staining above the optic disk. Left sensorineural hearing loss was confirmed by audiometry. Magnetic resonance imaging showed multiple areas of T_2-signal change (Figure). Enhancing perivascular lesions were seen bilaterally in the cerebral hemispheres and cerebellum. Cerebrospinal fluid analysis showed an increase in protein (114 mg/dL [normal, <45 mg/dL]) and cells (eight lymphocytes).

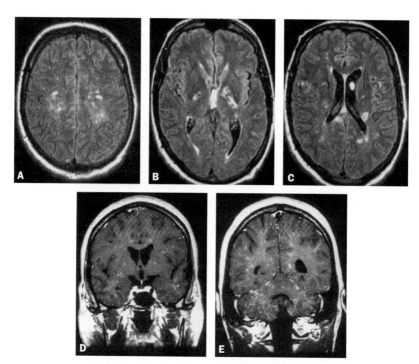

FIGURE. *A-C,* Axial T$_2$-weighted and, *D* and *E,* coronal T$_1$-weighted images with gadolinium enhancement showing multiple areas of T$_2$-signal increase and contrast enhancement in the cerebral hemispheres (periventricular region, internal capsule, basal ganglia, and corpus callosum) and left middle cerebellar peduncle. (*E* from Petty GW, Engel AG, Younge BR, *et al. Medicine (Baltimore)* 1998;**77**:12-40.)

Commentary by Dr. George W. Petty

Retinocochleocerebral vasculopathy (Susac's syndrome) is an acute or subacute syndrome of encephalopathy, visual loss, and hearing loss caused by multiple arteriolar occlusions in the brain, retina, and cochlea. Young adult women are afflicted more often than men, although patients as old as 51 years have been reported. The incidence is unknown. Although this syndrome is considered rare, it is likely encountered more often than it is recognized. Only a small proportion of the patients have the complete clinical triad at the onset of symptoms, making the initial diagnosis difficult. Patients with "partial" forms of the syndrome have been described (e.g., brain and retinal involvement without hearing loss). In many cases of Susac's syndrome, the initial diagnosis is multiple sclerosis, cardioembolic stroke, Ménière's disease, systemic lupus erythematosus, migraine, or schizophrenia.

Brain manifestations are protean and vary considerably. Some patients present with stroke-like episodes, whereas others have subacute dementia. Common manifestations include headache (often with migrainous features) and deficits in cognition, memory, language, and praxis. Behavior and affect are prominently involved, sometimes leading to psychiatric hospitalization. Gait disturbance due to a combination of cerebellar, corticospinal tract, and vestibular involvement is common. Corticospinal tract signs are frequently found on examination, but profound weakness and hemiplegia are uncommon. Sensory symptoms, sometimes fleeting, may simulate peripheral neuropathy.

The typical retinal manifestation is segmental visual loss in one or both eyes from retinal arteriolar occlusion. "Positive" migraine-like visual phenomena sometimes occur. In some patients, the arteriolar occlusions are so peripheral that no visual loss is experienced. Occasionally, patients may be so encephalopathic at the time of presentation that they are either unaware of or unable to report visual loss. Therefore, a dilated ophthalmoscopic examination of the retina by an ophthalmologist is often crucial for making the diagnosis.

Vestibulocochlear manifestations include tinnitus or hearing loss in one or both ears and vertigo. Because patients who are severely encephalopathic may not be able to participate in a bedside test of hearing, much less formal audiography, a collateral history suggesting recent hearing loss from family or friends can provide an important diagnostic clue.

Laboratory studies for procoagulant state, infection, and collagen vascular disease are usually nondiagnostic. Cerebrospinal fluid analysis may demonstrate a mild lymphocytic pleocytosis and increased protein level. Cerebral angiographic findings are usually normal. Magnetic resonance imaging of the brain shows multiple punctate areas of T_2-signal abnormality and enhancement in the gray and white matter. This frequently takes on a "miliary" pattern involving the cerebral and cerebellar hemispheres, corpus callosum, basal ganglia, thalami, and brainstem. The lesions are typically smaller and more numerous than those encountered in multiple sclerosis. Retinal examination shows arteriolar occlusion or narrowing, sometimes with "boxcar" segmentation of the blood within the vessels. Audiograms typically show low- to mid-frequency sensorineural hearing loss thought to be due to microvascular infarction of the cochlear apex.

The etiology of Susac's syndrome is unknown. Pathologic specimens from brain and muscle demonstrate small infarctions and perivascular lymphocytic infiltrates but not the fibrinoid necrosis typical of vasculitis. Pathologic evidence of muscle involvement as well as myalgias, arthralgias, and constitutional symptoms in some patients suggest that this is a systemic illness with a predilection for the brain, retina, and cochlea.

Because only a small number of patients have been reported, there is no treatment of established efficacy. Most reported patients have received various forms of immunosuppression. In recent years, some of the patients evaluated at Mayo Clinic appear to have had a favorable response to treatment with corticosteroids and either plasma exchange or intravenous immunoglobulin. In addition, antiplatelet agents such as aspirin may be given, but there is no apparent indication for anticoagulation.

The clinical course and outcome are variable. Most patients have a monophasic illness that lasts for months or years, although at least one patient with a late recurrence (18 years) has been reported. Frequently, the encephalopathy, visual loss, and hearing loss fluctuate or improve, permitting some patients to return to work. A small proportion of patients become bedridden, blind, and deaf.

REFERENCE

Petty GW, Engel AG, Younge BR, *et al.* Retinocochleocerebral vasculopathy. *Medicine (Baltimore)* 1998;**77**:12-40.

History

A 66-year-old woman presented with slowly progressive gait ataxia. Thirteen years ago, she noted that her "hamstrings felt tight." Ten years ago, she first noted loss of feeling in the left foot. The symptoms gradually worsened, involved the proximal leg, and then slowly became bilateral and symmetrical, involving both legs below the hips. Eight years ago, she noted poor balance while skiing and a feeling of numbness in the pelvic girdle bilaterally. Multiple neurologic evaluations failed to disclose a diagnosis. Her condition gradually worsened, and by the time of her evaluation at Mayo Clinic, she was unable to walk without holding on to furniture and her fingertips had recently lost feeling. She stated she did not have dry eyes or dry mouth. She had a past history of hypothyroidism and osteoporosis.

Examination

Neurologic examination demonstrated marked loss of vibration and proprioception and mild loss of temperature and pinprick sensations in the legs. There was no weakness. The deep tendon reflexes were reduced in the arms and absent in the legs. Finger-to-nose and heel-to-shin performance was reduced symmetrically. She had severe gait ataxia and a Romberg sign. She could not walk without touching the walls.

Investigations

Extensive studies for treatable forms of peripheral neuropathy were unrevealing. Nerve conduction studies (specifically, sural sensory nerve action potential [SNAP]) and electromyographic findings were normal. There was marked nonlocalized slowing of tibial somatosensory evoked potentials. Magnetic resonance imaging (MRI) showed thickened, enhancing nerve roots in the cauda equina (Figure 1). Cerebrospinal fluid analysis showed one cell and an increase in protein (103 mg/dL; normal, 14-45 mg/dL). A surgical procedure was performed.

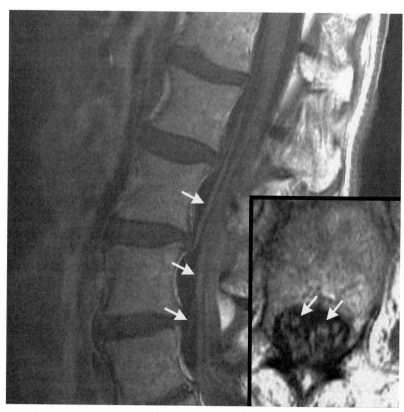

FIGURE 1. Sagittal and transverse (*inset*) T_1-weighted MRI of the cauda equina with gadolinium showing thickened and enhancing nerve roots (*arrows*).

Commentary by Drs. Michael Sinnreich and P. James B. Dyck

Several disorders present with sensory ataxia. Included in the pathogenesis are vitamin deficiencies, inherited degenerative conditions, infectious diseases, toxic substances, and inflammatory immune disorders. Sensory ataxia can be caused by varied involvement of the dorsal columns, dorsal root entry zone, dorsal root ganglia, and distal sensory axons. In our patient, peripheral sensory segments proximal to the dorsal root ganglia were affected, rendering the diagnosis of a peripheral nervous system disorder difficult because nerve conduction and electromyographic studies are normal. Thickened nerve roots seen on MRI and slowing of proprioceptive pathways from the lower extremities were helpful in localizing the lesion. A biopsy specimen from a fascicle of a lumbar nerve root showed edema, a marked decrease in the large-fiber population (with a shift to smaller diameter fibers), endoneurial inflammatory cells, and onion bulb formation (Figure 2). Despite the long duration of the patient's illness, the response to intravenous immunoglobulin treatment was rapid and substantial. After 16 weeks of first biweekly and then weekly intravenous immunoglobulin therapy, the patient had marked and quantifiable improvement. She could walk unaided and drive her car again, which was impossible before treatment because of proprioceptive impairment of the lower extremities. The acroparesthesias resolved.

Chronic immune demyelinating neuropathies can involve various segments of the peripheral nervous system. In classic chronic inflammatory demyelinating polyradiculoneuropathy (CIDP), proximal as well as distal nerve segments are affected, with predominant motor involvement. Certain paraprotein-associated demyelinating neuropathies may affect large sensory fibers in distal nerves. Multifocal motor neuropathy may involve motor fibers at multiple levels throughout the nerve. In Lewis-Sumner syndrome, sensory and motor fibers are involved multifocally in proximal and distal segments, predominantly in the upper extremities. This varied tropism has not been explained. Our patient has a different form of localized CIDP that involved peripheral sensory segments proximal to the dorsal root ganglia. The inflammatory immune pathogenesis is supported by 1) the increase in cerebrospinal fluid protein; 2) the rootlet biopsy findings of inflammatory cells, decreased number of large fibers, and onion bulb formation; and 3) the response to treatment.

Chronic immune sensory polyradiculopathy should be considered in the differential diagnosis of sensory ataxia because it is potentially treatable.

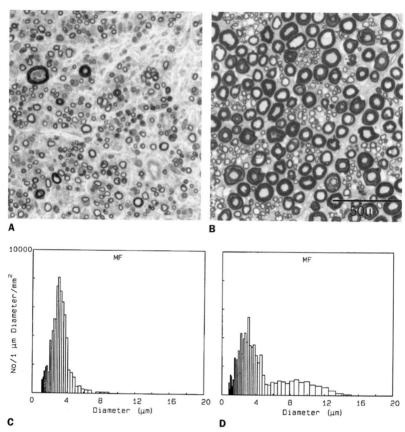

A   B

C   D

FIGURE 2. Comparison of biopsy specimen from lumbar rootlet of the patient (*A*) and an age-matched postmortem control (*B*) (see color insert). Note the markedly altered distribution of fiber size, with a decrease in the large-fiber population and normal fiber density in *A*. *C* and *D*, The respective myelinated fiber histograms show the patient's loss of Aαβ fibers.

REFERENCE

Sinnreich M, Daube JR, Klein CJ, *et al*. Inflammatory sensory polyradiculopathy (abstract). *Neurology* 2003;**60 Suppl 1**:A159.

History

A 20-year-old man was evaluated for long-standing cardiomyopathy. He was the product of a healthy pregnancy and birth. He achieved motor milestones normally throughout his childhood. At age 6, he was noted to have a learning disability and remained in special education classes until age 18. At age 16, he had episodes of reduced awareness and received treatment with anticonvulsants. At age 19, he had two witnessed generalized seizures. He was then noted to have asymptomatic cardiomegaly.

There was no history of alcohol use. The patient's two brothers died at ages 16 and 27 (the younger brother died of hypertrophic cardiomyopathy discovered at autopsy); one sister had findings of hypertrophic and dilated cardiomyopathy. Four other siblings were thought to be well, and the parents had no known heart disease.

Examination

The patient appeared moderately mentally retarded. The findings on neurologic examination were otherwise normal. The cardiac apex was displaced laterally, and a soft systolic murmur was present.

Investigations

The creatine kinase level was intermittently increased to twice the normal level (100% MM fraction). Extensive biochemical and hematologic studies were normal, as was urine myoglobin. The electroencephalogram was normal. Chest radiography demonstrated cardiomegaly, and electrocardiography documented first-degree heart block and left bundle branch block. Electromyography showed increased insertional activity in the sampled muscles and myotonic discharges in the paraspinal muscles. Echocardiography demonstrated hypertrophic cardiomyopathy with a reduced ejection fraction (46%). A diagnostic study was performed.

Cardioskeletal myopathy associated with lysosome-associated membrane protein-2 (LAMP-2) deficiency

Commentary by Dr. Duygu Selcen

The differential diagnosis in this case is hypertrophic cardioskeletal myopathy associated with mental retardation. Cardiomyopathies can be classified as hypertrophic, dilated, restrictive, and arrhythmogenic. In several disorders, they can be of more than one type, and in a given patient, they may change from one type to another. Cardiomyopathy can precede the onset of an associated skeletal muscle myopathy in some diseases, including Becker muscular dystrophy, Emery-Dreifuss muscular dystrophy, myotonic dystrophy, myofibrillar myopathy, acid maltase deficiency, and Danon disease. The associated mental retardation narrows the diagnosis to myotonic dystrophy and Danon disease.

Analysis of the skeletal muscle biopsy specimen was important in making the diagnosis in this case. Many muscle fibers in the triceps muscle harbored multiple small vacuoles, some surrounded by a blue halo in trichrome-stained sections (Figure). Because of their small size, the vacuoles were more apparent in 1-µm-thick resin sections. Histochemical studies showed acid phosphatase-positive material around and sometimes within the vacuoles. The overall glycogen content of muscle fibers was normal. In numerous muscle fibers, electron microscopy showed small membrane-bound autophagic vacuoles that contained miscellaneous cytoplasmic degradation products and small amounts of glycogen. These features were consistent with Danon disease and pointed away from the diagnosis of myotonic dystrophy. Immunostaining for LAMP-2 revealed the total absence of LAMP-2 in the muscle fibers. An immunoblot of the patient's muscle homogenate confirmed the absence of LAMP-2.

LAMP-2 is a lysosomal glycoprotein detected on lysosomal membranes and sometimes on the cell surface. It acts as a receptor for the selective import and degradation of cytosolic proteins in lysosomes and participates in chaperone-mediated autophagy. Targeted deletion of LAMP-2 in the mouse results in vacuolar changes in skeletal and cardiac muscle as well as in the liver and other organs, decreased cardiac contractility, and premature death.

In 1981, Danon et al. described "lysosomal glycogen storage disease with normal acid maltase" in two males who had proximal muscle weakness, cardiomyopathy, and mental retardation. Muscle biopsy studies revealed a vacuolar myopathy with excessive lysosomal activity and no acid maltase deficiency. Subsequent studies showed that some patients with Danon disease are not mentally retarded and some have hepatomegaly. In 2000, Nishino et al. discovered that Danon disease is caused by mutations in *LAMP2*, the gene at Xq24 that encodes LAMP-2. Affected females have milder disease and usually develop cardiac symptoms during middle age, but electrocardiography or echocardiography can demonstrate cardiac involvement even in the presymptomatic stage. Cardiac involvement in Danon disease is progressive, can change from a hypertrophic to a dilated form, and is fatal. Therefore, heart transplantation may be the most effective intervention in both affected males and females. Our patient died at age 23 despite having a pacemaker implanted as part of the management of his hypertrophic and dilated cardiomyopathy.

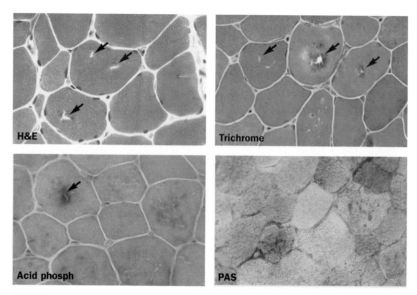

FIGURE. Note muscle fibers harboring multiple small vacuoles (*arrows*) surrounded by a halo of acid phosphatase positivity. Some vacuoles contain glycogen. H&E, hematoxylin and eosin; PAS, periodic acid-Schiff (see color insert). (Original magnification, x160.)

REFERENCES

Danon MJ, Oh SJ, DiMauro S, *et al*. Lysosomal glycogen storage disease with normal acid maltase. *Neurology* 1981;**31**:51-7.

Nishino I, Fu J, Tanji K, *et al*. Primary LAMP-2 deficiency causes X-linked vacuolar cardiomyopathy and myopathy (Danon disease). *Nature* 2000;**406**:906-10.

History

A 65-year-old man was evaluated for a 5-year history of a slowly progressive gait difficulty that was subacute in onset. He complained of stiffness of the lower limbs and difficulty with balance. Three years after the onset of gait difficulty, he began to use a cane and 1 year later, to use a walker. For 1 year before evaluation, he had paresthesias of the hands and feet. He also had a 5-year history of erectile dysfunction and a 1-year history of increased urinary frequency with urgency and hesitancy. His medications included aspirin and ranitidine. For the past 22 years, he had been taking 200 to 400 mg of zinc daily to prevent colds.

Examination

Neurologic examination demonstrated increased tone and mild weakness in the lower limbs, with an upper motor neuron pattern. He had difficulty on the heel-to-shin test. Rapid foot tapping was slow and clumsy. Vibration sensation in the lower limbs was impaired in a graded manner up to the knees, and position sense was impaired at the toes and malleoli. The reflexes were brisk except the ankle jerk, which was slightly depressed. The plantar response was extensor. He had a spastic-ataxic gait and was unable to walk tandemly. The Romberg test was positive.

Investigations

The following laboratory tests were normal: complete blood count, erythrocyte sedimentation rate, vitamin B_{12}, vitamin E, folate, iron, immunoelectrophoresis, thyroid-stimulating hormone, antinuclear antibody, electrolytes, liver enzymes, glucose, paraneoplastic panel, fatty acid profile, antiphospholipid antibody, lactate, amylase, and lipase. Serologic tests for syphilis, Lyme disease, human T-lymphocyte virus type I, and human immunodeficiency virus were unrevealing. The results of lumbar puncture were unremarkable except for a slight increase in protein concentration to 61 mg/dL. The urine heavy metal screening study (arsenic, lead, mercury, and cadmium) was normal. A nerve conduction study demonstrated a moderately severe axonal sensorimotor peripheral neuropathy. The median somatosensory evoked potentials showed slowing in the central pathways between the cervical spine and sensory cerebral cortex; the tibial response was absent. Magnetic resonance imaging (MRI) of the brain showed changes that could be attributed to small-vessel ischemic disease, and MRI of the cervical and lumbosacral spine showed degenerative disease-related changes not thought to be important. The serum level of ceruloplasmin was markedly decreased to 7.3 mg/dL (normal, 22.9-43.1 mg/dL) and the serum level of copper was reduced to 0.45 µg/mL (normal, 0.75-1.45 µg/mL). The serum level of zinc was increased at 1.51 µg/mL (normal, 0.66-1.10 µg/mL), and urine 24-hour zinc excretion was increased to 4,264 µg (normal, 300-600 µg). Urine 24-hour copper excretion was 22 µg (normal, 15-60 µg).

DIAGNOSIS CASE 33
Myeloneuropathy due to copper deficiency
(caused by chronic excessive oral intake of zinc)

Commentary by Dr. Neeraj Kumar

For more than two decades, the patient ingested 15 to 30 times the recommended daily allowance of zinc (recommended daily allowance, 15 mg). Neurologic examination was remarkable for spastic myelopathy and peripheral neuropathy. He stopped taking zinc and started receiving oral copper supplementation (copper, 2 mg/d). Six weeks later, the paresthesias had resolved and gait had improved markedly. The serum level of ceruloplasmin normalized to 32.5 mg/dL, as did serum copper (1.08 μg/mL). The serum level of zinc returned to normal at 0.95 μg/mL. The 24-hour copper excretion was again normal, and although 24-hour zinc excretion decreased markedly, it was still slightly elevated at 971 μg. The median somatosensory evoked potentials improved, and tibial evoked potentials were obtainable, albeit abnormal.

Copper is an essential trace metal and a component of many key metalloenzymes. Because the daily requirement is low and copper is widely available in foods, acquired copper deficiency in humans is rare. It can be seen with malnutrition, total parenteral nutrition, gastrectomy, or, as in our patient, excessive intake of zinc. Zinc interferes with the intestinal absorption of copper by inducing intestinal synthesis of metallothionein, an intracellular ligand (Figure). Copper has a higher affinity for metallothionein than zinc, displaces zinc from metallothionein, and is sequestered in enterocytes, which are then sloughed. This is the basis of zinc therapy in Wilson's disease.

Cytochrome-*c* oxidase is a copper-dependent enzyme required for iron uptake by mitochondria to form heme. In copper-deficient states, iron accumulates in the cytoplasm, forming sideroblasts. The commonest manifestations of acquired copper deficiency are anemia, neutropenia, and bone abnormalities. Unlike other patients reported in the literature, our patient did not have anemia.

Inherited copper deficiency (Menkes' disease) results in intellectual deterioration, failure to thrive, seizures, abnormal hair, and connective tissue abnormalities. Menkes' disease results from mutations in the *ATP7A* gene, which encodes a copper-transporting P-type ATPase. Even though Wilson's disease is a disorder of copper excess, the mutated gene (*ATP7B*) is a close homologue of *ATP7A* and encodes a P-type ATPase that is highly expressed in the liver and is a close homologue of the gene product for Menkes' disease. Dietary copper deficiency in ruminants, "swayback disease," results in progressive myelopathy and ataxia. The literature on the neurologic manifestations of acquired copper deficiency in humans is limited. The first report was that of Schleper and Stuerenburg in 2001, who described a 46-year-old woman who presented with an 18-month history of progressive spastic tetraparesis, ataxic gait, and paresthesias. Prodan et al. recently reported on two patients with idiopathic hyperzincemia and hypocupremia who, on MRI, had evidence of central nervous system demyelination. Also, a cluster of patients who had multiple sclerosis and were associated with a manufacturing industry that used zinc as a principal raw material has been reported. An increased plasma level of zinc has also been described as a heritable anomaly with no clinical manifestations. Few reports are available on the appropriate dose and route of copper replacement therapy. There has been concern that the elimination of zinc may be slow, and until such elimination occurs, the intestinal absorption of copper is blocked.

Hereditary aceruloplasminemia is a newly recognized disorder of iron metabolism that has been associated with ataxia, retinal degeneration, blepharospasm, and basal ganglia degeneration. Ceruloplasmin is a major source of plasma ferroxidase activity and is important in protecting neurons against oxidative stress associated with iron metabolism. Hereditary ceruloplasmin deficiency has been shown to increase advanced glycation end products in the brain. Menkes' disease and swayback disease are associated with defective oxidative phosphorylation, with decreased activity of cytochrome oxidase. Defective oxidative phosphorylation caused by mitochondrial iron overload occurs in Friedreich's ataxia. Wilson's disease is associated with the accumulation of intracellular iron and copper. Impaired mitochondrial metabolism possibly represents the final common pathway for neuronal injury in these disorders.

Clinicians should be vigilant to the signs of myelopathy or neuropathy in patients at risk for copper deficiency. Caution should be exercised in taking large doses of "over-the-counter" zinc. Prompt recognition is essential to prevent progressive deterioration. The determination of ceruloplasmin levels should be included in the work-up of patients with myelopathy of unclear origin.

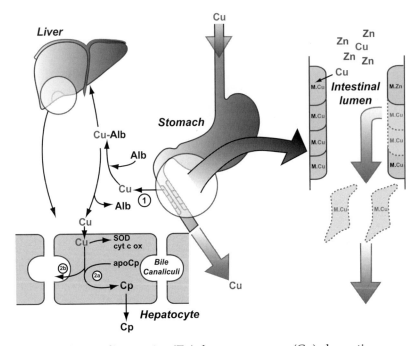

FIGURE. Excess dietary zinc (Zn) decreases copper (Cu) absorption by inducing metallothionein (M) formation in mucosal cells. Metallothioneins have a high affinity for Cu and bind it preferentially. The bound Cu is lost as the cells slough into the intestinal lumen. By this mucosal block, Zn induces a negative Cu balance. Failure to mobilize absorbed Cu from intestinal cells is the basis of Menkes' disease ((1)). In Wilson's disease, there is decreased incorporation of Cu into ceruloplasmin (Cp) ((2a)) and impaired biliary excretion of Cu ((2b)). Alb, albumin; apoCp, apolipoprotein ceruloplasmin; cyt c ox, cytochrome-*c* oxidase; SOD, superoxide dismutase (see color insert).

REFERENCE

Kumar N, Gross JB Jr, Ahlskog JE. Myelopathy due to copper deficiency. *Neurology* 2003;**61**:273-4.

History

A 73-year-old man complained of a 1-year history of numbness of the cheek that developed after a senile keratosis had been removed. For 10 months, he experienced both constant and stabbing pain in the left cheek; later, the pain involved the left pinna and neck. He noted weakness first of the forehead and eyebrow and then of the angle of the mouth and grimacing muscles. Vision, chewing, and swallowing were normal. He had an 8-year history of benign positional vertigo. Magnetic resonance imaging (MRI) of the skull base reportedly showed no abnormality.

Examination

All facial muscles on the left, including the platysma, were severely weak. He could wiggle his ears bilaterally. Tear production, the afferent corneal response, nasal tickle, and taste appeared to be normal. Pinprick sensation was reduced along the maxillary division of the left trigeminal nerve. There were no palpable masses in the neck.

Investigations

Computed tomographic (CT) findings of the skull base were normal. MRI demonstrated faint gadolinium enhancement of the facial nerve in the left middle ear cavity. At surgery, a peripheral branch and the main trunk of the facial nerve were normal. A branch of the superior division of the buccal nerve appeared scarred and inflamed.

Commentary by Dr. Raymond G. Auger

The patient presented with a progressive disorder of the facial nerve caused by neoplastic infiltration of its perineural sheath (Figure). Nests of high-grade squamous carcinoma cells were found within the buccal nerve in this case. This case demonstrates the need to consider extracranial involvement of the facial nerve in patients presenting with facial weakness.

The site of the lesion causing facial paresis in a patient can be deduced clinically by assessing the presence or absence of lacrimation (greater superficial petrosal nerve), hyperacusis (nerve to the stapedius muscle), and taste (chorda tympani). In this patient, taste was normal, suggesting that the lesion was distal to the junction of the chorda tympani and the main trunk of the facial nerve. The patient volunteered the information that he was able to wiggle his ears bilaterally. This was of localizing significance because the branch to the posterior auricular muscle is the first branch of the facial nerve after it exits the stylomastoid foramen. Therefore, the observation that this muscle was normal despite the severe weakness of the other muscles supplied by the facial nerve provided irrefutable evidence that the lesion was in the extracranial portion of the facial nerve.

The other relevant feature of the patient's history is the evolution of the facial weakness, which began in the upper portion of the face and, over several weeks, spread to lower portions of the face. This pattern of involvement indicates that the various branches of the facial nerve were involved at different times. In contrast, when the intracranial portion of the facial nerve is involved, the peripheral manifestations are usually distributed more uniformly among the different branches of the nerve.

The most common tumor that can present in this fashion is adenoid cystic carcinoma of the parotid gland. It may cause severe involvement of the facial nerve through perineural spread. Frequently, a palpable mass is not present, and MRI or CT may not detect the tumor. When confronted with this presentation, exploratory surgery by a head and neck surgeon should be recommended. In our patient, surgery confirmed the presence of a high-grade squamous cell carcinoma that invaded the perineural sheath.

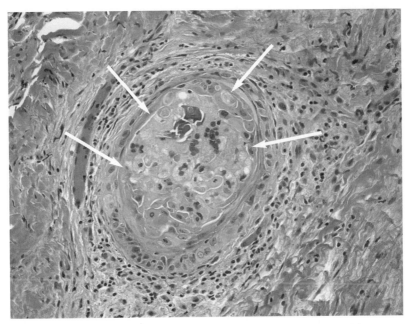

FIGURE. A branch of the facial nerve (*arrows*) has been replaced by high-grade squamous cell carcinoma (see color insert). (Hematoxylin-eosin stain; original magnification, x200.)

REFERENCES

Broderick JP, Auger RG, DeSanto LW. Facial paralysis and occult parotid cancer: a characteristic syndrome. *Arch Otolaryngol Head Neck Surg* 1988;**114**:195-7.

Clement P, Rondet P, Marlier F, *et al.* Isolated facial palsy and occult adenoid cystic carcinoma of the parotid [French]. *Ann Otolaryngol Chir Cervicofac* 2001;**118**:61-3.

History

A 25-year-old man has had seizures since early childhood. At age 2 years, he was in a postictal coma for several hours until he received treatment for profound hypoglycemia. He remained comatose for 2 weeks thereafter and was blind bilaterally until his sight recovered 6 weeks later. Recurrent generalized seizures preceded by a brief aura of "rainbow lights" were imperfectly controlled with multiple antiepileptic medications. Since childhood, he also has had severe orthostatic intolerance with syncope, and his teacher stood behind him in the lunch line to catch him when he fell. Recently, despite treatment with high doses of fludrocortisone, he could stand no longer than a few moments without collapsing or squatting. He described nasal stuffiness, incapacitating daytime fatigue, and enuresis requiring an external catheter at night. He reported normal sweating in response to heat. He was thought to be learning-disabled. A brother had been stillborn.

Examination

Blood pressure decreased severely upon standing. The distal hands and central face were hypoplastic. Pupillary reactions were normal, but eye movements were saccadic, and he had mild appendicular and gait ataxia.

Investigations

The electroencephalogram was normal. Magnetic resonance imaging of the brain showed sinus opacification, but otherwise the findings were normal. Autonomic testing demonstrated severe orthostatic hypotension with preserved compensatory tachycardia (Figure). Adrenergic components of the Valsalva maneuver were absent, whereas the Valsalva ratio and tests of sudomotor function were normal. Plasma norepinephrine was undetectable at <10 pg/mL (normal, 70-750 pg/mL), as was epinephrine at <10 pg/mL (normal, undetectable to 110 pg/mL). Plasma dopamine, by contrast, was elevated at 35 pg/mL (normal, <30 pg/mL).

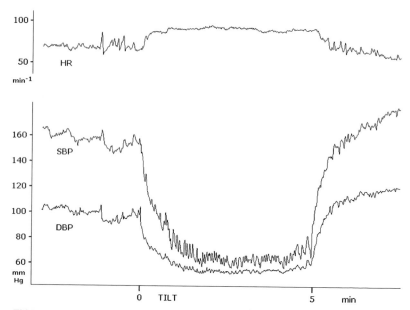

FIGURE. Tilt table test at 80° for 5 minutes shows beat-to-beat heart rate (HR) and systolic (SBP) and diastolic (DBP) blood pressure responses. Syncope did not occur. Note profound orthostatic hypotension with preserved compensatory tachycardia.

Commentary by Dr. William P. Cheshire

Norepinephrine, the principal sympathetic neurotransmitter, is synthesized within the chromaffin granules of the adrenal medulla and the synaptic vesicles of noradrenergic neurons from dopamine by DBH. Congenital DBH deficiency, a rare disorder, was first recognized in 1986 by Robertson et al. in the United States and Man in't Velt et al. in the Netherlands. Immunohistochemical studies of perivascular cutaneous tissue have shown structurally intact sympathetic nerve terminals lacking DBH immunoreactivity, consistent with an enzymatic defect. Molecular genetic analysis of several families has revealed a heterogeneous variety of mutations in the DBH gene on chromosome 9, with a recessive pattern of inheritance. The high incidence of spontaneous abortions and stillbirths among parents of afflicted persons suggests that mutations in the DBH gene can endanger fetal survival.

Because norepinephrine is essential for the peripheral vascular constriction that normally maintains blood pressure in response to blood volume redistribution upon standing, DBH deficiency is characterized by severe orthostatic hypotension that presents in childhood. Orthostatic collapse or syncope can be mistaken for epileptic seizures and is not prevented by antiepileptic medications. Also, because norepinephrine is the precursor of epinephrine, which is required for glycogenolysis and thermogenesis, patients are subject to episodic hypoglycemia and hypothermia, particularly during the first year after birth. Additional clinical features typically include exercise-induced hypotension, fatigue, altered mentation, nasal stuffiness, ptosis, brachydactyly, nocturia, and retrograde ejaculation. Cognitive function is normal, although hypotension can impair attention and vigilance. Nocturia may be due to the natriuretic effect of excessive dopamine. Some patients have hyperextensible joints, mild facial weakness, and hypotonic skeletal muscles.

DBH deficiency can be distinguished clinically from most forms of generalized autonomic failure by the congenital onset of symptoms dominated by disabling orthostatic hypotension and by sympathetic dysfunction that is localized exclusively to the noradrenergic system. Parasympathetic and sympathetic cholinergic functions, for example, are spared. Accordingly, clinical autonomic testing in this case showed profound adrenergic failure but preserved sympathetic cholinergic sudomotor function. Parasympathetic function was intact also, as shown by normal heart rate variability to deep breathing and the Valsalva maneuver and by normal tachycardia in response to orthostatic hypotension. The finding unique to DBH deficiency was the virtual absence of circulating levels of norepinephrine and epinephrine in combination with increased levels of the precursor dopamine.

Patients with DBH deficiency do not respond to standard pharmacologic treatments for orthostatic hypotension. Effective treatment consists of bypassing the enzymatic defect with L-threo-3,4-dihydroxyphenylserine (DOPS), an amino acid that is decarboxylated directly to norepinephrine by L-aromatic amino acid decarboxylase. Administered orally, DOPS dramatically restores blood pressure and circulating levels of norepinephrine. In our patient, the symptoms of orthostatic hypotension resolved almost completely after treatment with DOPS was initiated.

REFERENCE

Vincent S, Robertson D. The broader view: catecholamine abnormalities. *Clin Auton Res* 2002;**12 Suppl 1**:44-9.

History

Two years before evaluation at Mayo Clinic (Jacksonville), a 57-year-old man developed headaches, blurred vision, and obscurations of vision and had been told that he had papilledema. He noted progressive fatigue, tinnitus, bilateral hearing loss, and paresthesias of both feet and, later, both hands. Previous computed tomographic and magnetic resonance imaging scans of the brain were normal, and cerebrospinal fluid analysis demonstrated an increased protein concentration (twice normal) and an elevated opening pressure (190 mm H_2O). At the Mayo evaluation, he complained that his lower extremities below the knees and his distal arms were numb and burning. Also, impotence, general malaise, diffuse weakness, darkening of his skin, and whitening of his fingernails and toenails had developed.

Examination

General physical examination demonstrated enlarged cervical lymph nodes, hyperpigmentation of the skin diffusely, angiomas of the skin diffusely, pedal edema, white fingernails and toenails, purplish discoloration of the fingers, gynecomastia, and hepatomegaly. On ophthalmologic examination, visual acuity was 20/20 in both eyes and bilateral optic disk edema was noted. Neurologic examination showed markedly decreased hearing bilaterally, marked gait instability, and a severe sensorimotor peripheral polyneuropathy affecting all sensory modalities, with sensory levels at the upper thighs and mid-arms bilaterally.

Investigations

Lumbar puncture revealed an opening pressure of 240 mm H_2O, with cerebrospinal fluid contents normal except for a protein level of 118 mg/dL. Endocrine studies demonstrated decreased total and free testosterone, increased prolactin, mild hypoadrenalism, and hypothyroidism. Serum immunoelectrophoresis showed an abnormal IgG λ protein, and urine immunoelectrophoresis revealed a monoclonal λ protein plus an IgG λ fragment. A solitary sclerotic lesion in the first lumbar segment was found on a bone survey, and magnetic resonance imaging showed that the lesion was an enhancing mass that invaded vertebra L1 and extended into the right paravertebral soft tissue (Figure). Lymph node and bone marrow biopsies were performed.

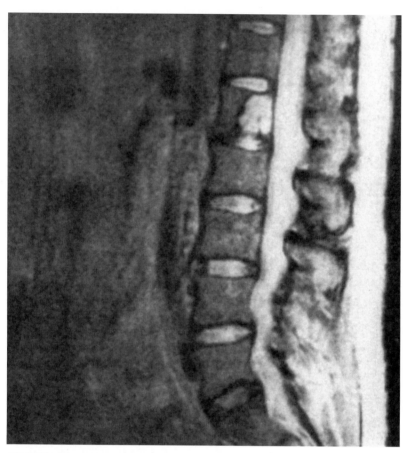

FIGURE. Magnetic resonance T$_2$-weighted image showing a hyperintense focus in the posterior aspect of vertebral body L1. (From Bolling JP, Brazis PW. *Am J Ophthalmol* 1990;**109:**503-10. By permission of Elsevier.)

Commentary by Dr. Paul W. Brazis

The lymph node and bone marrow biopsy findings were consistent with Castleman's disease, and a bone marrow biopsy specimen showed only a slight increase in the number of plasma cells. POEMS syndrome is a multisystem disorder of patients with monoclonal gammopathy. The osteosclerotic form of myeloma seems to be strongly associated with POEMS syndrome in that 85% of patients with this syndrome have either osteosclerotic or mixed osteosclerotic and lytic forms, although the osteosclerotic variant accounts for only 1% to 2% of cases of multiple myeloma.

Peripheral neuropathy is the major component of POEMS syndrome and is usually progressive, motor or sensorimotor in type, and present in virtually all patients. Endocrine abnormalities are found in 60% to 80% of patients and include gynecomastia and impotence, glucose intolerance or diabetes, hypothyroidism or hyperthyroidism, and adrenal insufficiency. The most common skin change is diffuse hyperpigmentation, noted in more than 90% of patients. Apparent thickening of the skin and hypertrichosis also occur. Hepatomegaly is the most common organomegaly (82% of patients). Splenomegaly and lymphadenopathy are also common, with histopathologic findings on lymph node biopsy usually indicative of Castleman's disease. Other, less common findings with POEMS syndrome include peripheral edema, pleural effusion, finger clubbing, white fingernails and toenails, ascites, fever, verrucous angiomas, and pupillary light-near dissociation.

Optic disk swelling is noted in approximately two-thirds of patients. Its cause is unclear because many patients have normal lumbar puncture opening pressures.

For patients who have a single localized sclerotic lesion (as in the patient presented here), radiation or surgical extirpation, occasionally in combination with chemotherapy, may improve the condition or even induce complete remission. Patients with multiple osteosclerotic lesions may have a response to chemotherapy, but it is usually poor compared with that of patients with a single plasmacytoma. The patient's condition has stabilized, and he is doing reasonably well now 5 years after diagnosis, although he is significantly disabled by the peripheral polyneuropathy.

REFERENCE

Bolling JP, Brazis PW. Optic disk swelling with peripheral neuropathy, organomegaly, endocrinopathy, monoclonal gammopathy, and skin changes (POEMS syndrome). *Am J Ophthalmol* 1990;**109**:503-10.

History

A 56-year-old man developed subacute numbness, tingling, and weakness on the left side of his face, followed by progressive dysarthria, increasing headache, bilateral hearing loss, nocturnal confusion, hiccups, and increasingly severe truncal and left limb ataxia. Within 12 weeks, he was confined to bed and was unable to stand and walk because of the ataxia. He did not appear to have a response to a 1-week trial of oral prednisone therapy.

Examination

He was fully oriented. Counterclockwise rotatory nystagmus was noted on right gaze and horizontal nystagmus on left gaze. Neurologic examination also demonstrated left lower motor neuron facial weakness, bilateral hearing loss, Horner's syndrome on the left, and ataxic dysarthria. He had severe truncal and left limb ataxia and a Babinski sign on the right.

Investigations

Cerebrospinal fluid analysis showed 20 leukocytes (88% lymphocytes), an increase in protein (103 mg/dL [normal, 14-45 mg/dL]), normal glucose, and no oligoclonal bands. The results of cytologic study were negative. Serial magnetic resonance imaging (MRI) studies showed progressive changes of increased T_2 signal in the corpus callosum, left frontal lobe, right cerebral peduncle, left brachium pontis, pons, and ventral brainstem, with mass effect on the fourth ventricle (Figure). Contrast enhancement was seen within the brainstem, periventricular white matter, and right cerebral peduncle. A diagnostic procedure was performed.

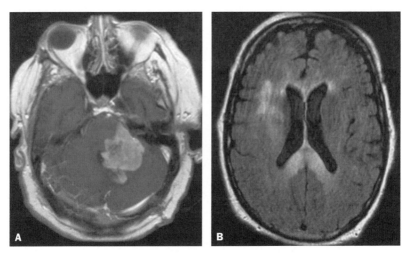

FIGURE. *A*, T$_1$-weighted MRI with gadolinium showing extension of signal abnormality with contrast enhancement in the left brachium pontis and left cerebral peduncle, with distortion of the fourth ventricle. *B*, Axial FLAIR MRI showing abnormal T$_2$ signal consistent with transcallosal involvement.

Commentary by Dr. Irene Meissner

The patient presented with a subacute progressive process that occurred over several months and affected cognition, multiple cranial nerves, and sympathetic, cerebellar, and pyramidal tracts, with associated imaging abnormalities. The symptoms of subtle cognitive changes, hearing loss (superimposed on known occupational hearing deficits), and multifocal white matter changes can be seen in many disorders. These include demyelinating processes, inflammatory disorders such as the microangiopathy of Susac's syndrome (retinocochleocerebral vestibulopathy), sarcoidosis, Behçet's syndrome, *Listeria* rhombencephalitis, and infiltrative tumors such as lymphoma or gliomatosis cerebri. In our patient, a brain biopsy specimen contained tumor cells positive for CD20 and CD79a, with a κ light chain restriction supporting the diagnosis of diffuse B-cell lymphoma (PCNSL).

The clinical diagnosis of PCNSL can be challenging, particularly because of the increased risk of this tumor associated with connective tissue diseases such as Sjögren's syndrome and inflammatory disorders such as systemic lupus erythematosus—diseases that can simulate PCNSL. Also, it is more common in chronic immunosuppression (cardiac, thymic, and renal transplantation) and immunodeficiency syndromes, including acquired immunodeficiency syndrome. Several other uncommon neurologic syndromes in patients with PCNSL that should raise the possibility of this diagnosis include uveocyclitis, subacute encephalitis with subependymal infiltration, and multiple sclerosis–like illness with a relapsing-remitting course.

Previously, PCNSL was thought to be a rare tumor, but its incidence has increased by a factor of 7 to 10 in the past two decades in both immunocompromised and immunocompetent populations. Epstein-Barr virus likely has an etiologic role in the immunocompromised form, but the cause of the immunocompetent form, as in our patient, is not known.

The clinical presentation of PCNSL includes focal symptoms (hemimotor, hemisensory, visual field deficits, brainstem or cerebellar signs, aphasia, seizures) or generalized signs (increased intracranial pressure, dementia, encephalopathy). The duration of symptoms from the onset to diagnosis is typically 3 months.

Computed tomography and MRI typically show isolated or multiple periventricular, homogeneously enhancing lesions, but atypical features such as ringlike enhancement can simulate inflammatory or infectious lesions. In the majority of cases, the lesions are lobar (hemispheric gray and adjacent white matter), with one-fourth of the lesions located in deep midline structures (septum pellucidum, basal ganglia, or corpus callosum). Most PCNSLs contact either the ependymal or meningeal surface or both, suggesting a meningioma (pseudomeningioma pattern). However, the lack of calcification and the tendency toward multiplicity favor PCNSL. The spontaneous (or steroid-induced) disappearance of lesions is classic, hence the term "ghost tumor."

Diagnosis is dependent on pathologic study, which shows malignant large cell diffuse B-cell lymphomas in 80% to 90% of patients. Detection of lymphomatous cells in the cerebrospinal or vitreous fluid (10%-20% of patients) can obviate cerebral biopsy. The role of surgery is restricted to diagnostic biopsy because of the multifocal, diffuse nature of the tumor and because the patients generally are elderly.

The prognosis for patients with PCNSL is grim, with a median survival of less than 2 years; the 5-year survival rate is less than 5%. Debate continues about the optimal dose of irradiation and the combination of methotrexate-based chemotherapy and radiation because of the neurotoxic effects of progressive leukoencephalopathy and cognitive dysfunction, particularly in the elderly. Cerebral recurrence is common, with a median survival of 12 to 18 months for patients treated with whole-brain radiation alone. Several phase II studies have shown substantial improvement in median survival (23-42 months) with combination methotrexate and radiation regimens. More recent studies have used methotrexate chemotherapy alone (delaying radiotherapy in patients who had a response to chemotherapy), with promising results.

Alternative strategies to improve the effectiveness of chemotherapy are being studied, including intra-arterial chemotherapy with osmotic blood-brain barrier disruption or intensive chemotherapy with hematopoietic stem-cell rescue.

REFERENCE

Olson JE, Janney CA, Rao RD, *et al*. The continuing increase in the incidence of primary central nervous system non-Hodgkin lymphoma: a surveillance, epidemiology, and end results analysis. *Cancer* 2002;**95**:1504-10.

History

A 68-year-old woman had a 1-year history of recurring stereotypic spells approximately twice monthly. They typically occurred in the evening while she was quietly watching television. She noted gradually worsening blurring of vision in the left eye such that within 15 minutes she had no meaningful vision. At about this time, she also noticed a moderately severe, steady discomfort within and around the left globe which spread to involve the ipsilateral forehead and temporal region, possibly with some associated mild increase in tearing. If she remained sitting upright, two 500-mg acetaminophen tablets would allow her to nap for 30 minutes, by which time her spell would have resolved completely. She avoided lying down, certain that this change in posture would worsen her symptoms. She had a past medical history of well-treated renovascular hypertension.

Examination

The findings on neurologic examination were normal.

Investigations

The erythrocyte sedimentation rate was 33 mm/h (normal, 0-29 mm/h). Magnetic resonance imaging (MRI) showed extensive focal and patchy chronic small-vessel ischemic changes in the perivascular white matter, old left basal ganglia lacunar infarcts, and basilar artery ectasia. The results of magnetic resonance angiography were essentially normal. A diagnostic study was performed.

Commentary by Dr. Jerry W. Swanson

Although transient monocular visual loss lasting minutes has several causes, including ischemia of the retina or optic nerve, related to different processes and intraocular conditions, the diagnosis of acute intermittent angle-closure glaucoma can be suspected on the basis of the history and confirmed on examination (Figure). On slit-lamp examination, the patient was found to have shallow anterior chambers. Baseline intraocular pressure was normal (16 mm Hg) but increased in the left eye to 32 mm Hg after dilatation with tropicamide 0.5%.

Acute angle-closure glaucoma occurs with apposition or adhesion (or both) of the iris to the trabecular meshwork, causing a decrease in the outflow of aqueous humor and an increase in intraocular pressure to high levels. Acute-angle closure is the sudden, circumferential, iridotrabecular apposition that causes a rapid, severe, and symptomatic rise in intraocular pressure. Symptoms of acute angle-closure glaucoma include blurred vision (from corneal edema), often with "halos" around lights, and pain, which can be severe, localized to the eye or radiating to the teeth, ear, sinuses, and forehead. Nausea and vomiting may occur. Episodes may be precipitated by dilatation of the pupil from physiologic events such as entering a darkened environment or pharmacologic mechanisms with mydriatic eyedrops or systemic drugs that cause mydriasis. Intermittent angle-closure glaucoma occurs with self-limited episodes of iridotrabecular apposition; the signs and symptoms are milder than in acute angle-closure glaucoma, as in our patient.

Factors that increase the risk of angle-closure glaucoma include a positive family history for angle closure, age older than 40 to 50 years, female sex, hyperopia, pseudoexfoliation, and racial group (Eskimo>Asian>African=white).

Signs of acute angle-closure glaucoma include a red eye with ciliary and conjunctival injection, tearing, eyelid edema, a cloudy-appearing cornea due to edema, a dilated unresponsive pupil caused by ischemia of the pupillary sphincter, and marked increase in intraocular pressure. During an attack of acute angle-closure glaucoma, the optic nerve head may be swollen and hyperemic. A narrow-angle configuration and shallow anterior chamber are usually present on examination, even between attacks.

Treatment includes miotic agents to acutely lower increased intraocular pressure. Laser iridotomy is the usual definitive treatment. This procedure eliminates the difference in pressure between the anterior and posterior chambers and alleviates the iris convexity.

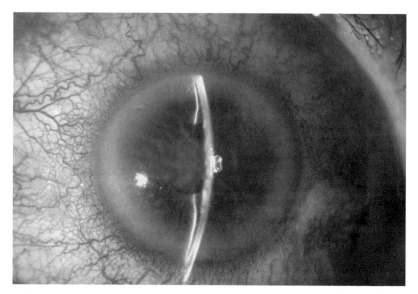

FIGURE. Acute angle-closure glaucoma. Note injection of globe, steamy cornea, and slit beam, which demonstrates narrow angles (see color insert).

REFERENCE

Yanoff M, Duker JS, Augsburger JJ, *et al*, Eds. *Ophthalmology*. London: Mosby; 1999.

History

A 39-year-old man noticed reduced dexterity at age 14 years. His symptoms progressed and within 9 months a profound tremor had developed that involved both the trunk and extremities. The tremor was worsened by activity but was also present at rest. His face and voice were spared. He noted that alcohol partially reduced the tremor. Several medications, including phenytoin, diazepam, benztropine, diphenhydramine, methazolamide, and carbidopa/levodopa, failed to reduce the tremor. He was not of Jewish ancestry and did not have a family history of consanguinity. His father had Parkinson's disease, and dystonia had been diagnosed in two sisters, one of whom had died early in childhood; two brothers were apparently healthy.

Examination

Neurologic examination demonstrated the following: voice tremor, marked truncal tremor, scoliosis, phasic torticollis, hypertrophy of the sternocleidomastoid muscle bilaterally, and dystonia of the trunk and left arm and leg. The fundus was normal, as was the rest of the examination.

Investigations

Findings on magnetic resonance imaging (MRI) of the brain were unremarkable. Surface electromyography of multiple proximal and distal arm muscles demonstrated motor unit grouping at 6 Hz in the bilateral wrist flexors, wrist extensors, and hand muscles when the arms were outstretched but not at rest, consistent with essential tremor or dystonia. The results of previous blood tests, including a chemistry panel, thyroid function test, complete blood count, smear for acanthocytes, and serum ceruloplasmin, were all normal.

DIAGNOSIS CASE 39
Hereditary generalized dystonia and tremor
secondary to *DYT1* gene mutation

Commentary by Drs. Charles H. Adler and Manfred D. Muenter

Patients with childhood- or adolescent-onset dystonia or tremor (or both) often have a hereditary disorder. Our patient's family history of Parkinson's disease in the father (not evaluated by us) and dystonia in two of four siblings suggested a possible autosomal dominant disorder.

DYT-1 dystonia is the most common cause of hereditary, autosomal dominantly inherited dystonia (Table). It is usually characterized by a generalized dystonia that often begins in the lower limbs and progresses over a few years. In some patients only a focal dystonia, usually of the arm, develops. Facial or cervical dystonia at disease onset is extremely rare, and relatively few patients ever have facial dystonia. However, the expression within a family is variable, and the phenomenology may be different in the anatomical location or severity of the dystonia. Also, the penetrance of this disorder is reduced, and dystonia develops in only about 30% of persons who inherit the mutation. The average age at onset is 13 years, and almost all patients have disease onset by age 26. Although this mutation has been found in multiple ethnic groups (accounting for 30% to 40% of cases of early-onset dystonia in non-Jewish populations), the occurrence is high in the Ashkenazi Jewish population (accounting for up to 80% of cases of early-onset dystonia).

The *DYT1* gene is located on chromosome 9 (9q34). Two mutations have been identified: a GAG (glutamic acid) deletion and a six–amino acid deletion. A test is commercially available to detect these deletions. Any patient with early-onset dystonia (or tremor), especially those with limb-onset or generalized dystonia, should have genetic counseling and have a blood sample tested for a *DYT1* deletion.

The pathophysiology of DYT-1 dystonia is not known. However, it is known that the gene codes for the protein torsin-A, which is an ATP-binding protein, but the function of this protein is unclear. Torsin-A is abundant in the dopaminergic neurons in the substantia nigra pars compacta, cerebellum, and hippocampus. However, how this mutation results in abnormal involuntary movements is unclear. Neuropathology and neurochemical studies have not demonstrated a cause.

Although DYT-1 dystonia was highly likely in our patient, it was important to evaluate for other causes because he did not have Jewish ancestry. An important autosomal recessive inherited dystonia is dopa-responsive dystonia (DRD). Multiple mutations have been found in genes that code for proteins with a role in dopamine synthesis (GTP cyclohydrolase I, tyrosine hydroxylase). Currently, no genetic test for this disorder is commercially available. However, as with our patient, it is important to try treating early-onset dystonia with levodopa. Levodopa can be almost "curative" in these patients because it is converted to dopamine by dopa decarboxylase and most patients have an almost complete, long-lasting (decades) response to a low dose.

Currently, no cure is available for DYT-1 dystonia. For patients with generalized dystonia, trials of anticholinergics, baclofen, anticonvulsants, or benzodiazepines have sometimes been successful. It is important to start at a low dose and very gradually titrate the dose upward. Focal dystonia, or even generalized dystonia that affects one or two regions most severely, may be treated with injections of botulinum toxin. This treatment can be just as successful for nonhereditary focal dystonia. Recent data have shown that deep-brain stimulation surgery, similar to that used for essential tremor and Parkinson's disease, is effective in some patients with DYT-1 generalized dystonia. The U.S. Food and Drug Administration has approved deep-brain stimulation for the treatment of DYT-1 generalized dystonia.

Table Identification and Characterization of Various Forms of Hereditary Dystonia

Dystonia type	Designation	Clinical signs	Mode	Chromosome	Gene abnormality
DYT-1	Early-onset generalized TD	Limb first, then generalizes	AD	9q34	Deletions in torsin A; test commercially available
DYT-2	AR, TD	Early-onset, generalized or segmental TD	AR	Unknown	Unknown
DYT-3	X-linked dystonia and parkinsonism, Lubag	Generalized or segmental TD ± parkinsonism	XR	Xq13.1	Unknown
DYT-4	Whispering dysphonia	Dystonia of larynx and other regions	AD	Unknown	Unknown
DYT-5a	Dopa-responsive dystonia	Dystonia with some parkinsonism	AD	14q22	Mutation of GTP cyclohydrolase I
DYT-5b	Dopa-responsive dystonia	Dystonia with some parkinsonism	AR	11p15.5	Mutation of tyrosine hydroxylase
DYT-6	Adolescent-onset TD	Mostly segmental dystonia	AD	8p21-22	Unknown

Table (continued)

Dystonia type	Designation	Clinical signs	Mode	Chromosome	Gene abnormality
DYT-7	Adult-onset focal dystonia	All types of focal dystonia	AD	18p	Unknown
DYT-8	PDC or paroxysmal non-kinesiogenic dyskinesia	Short attacks of dystonia, chorea precipitated by stress, alcohol, fatigue	AD	2q33-q25	Unknown
DYT-9	PDC with episodic ataxia/spasticity	Same as for PDC plus spastic paraplegia between attacks	AD	1p21-p13.3	Candidate gene: K+ channel gene KCNA3
DYT-10	Paroxysmal kinesiogenic choreoathetosis	Movements cause dystonia and choreic attacks	AD	16p11.2-q12.1	Unknown
DYT-11	Myoclonic-dystonia	Myoclonus plus dystonia responsive to alcohol	AD	7q21;11q23	Mutation in ε-sarcoglycan; dopamine D2 receptor gene change

Table (continued)

Dystonia type	Designation	Clinical signs	Mode	Chromosome	Gene abnormality
DYT-12	Rapid-onset dystonia/parkinsonism	Acute, subacute generalized dystonia and parkinsonism	AD	19q13	Unknown
DYT-13	Early-/adult-onset cranial, cervical, brachial	Onset by age 40; mainly focal dystonia	AD	1p36	Unknown

AD, autosomal dominant; AR, autosomal recessive; PDC, paroxysmal dystonic choreoathetosis; TD, torsion dystonia; XR, X-linked recessive.

REFERENCE

Klein C, Ozelius LJ. Dystonia: clinical features, genetics, and treatment. *Curr Opin Neurol* 2002;**15**:491-7.

History

A 51-year-old man had a 33-year history of recurrent headaches with hemiplegia. Approximately six times each year, scintillating scotoma, photophobia, and nausea developed, followed by a severe, throbbing, unilateral left-sided headache, right-sided hemisensory loss, and hemiplegia that would resolve within 6 days. Other family members experienced similar episodes. Within the last several years, his family noted a personality change. He seemed depressed. Concerned family members brought him to the hospital when they found him lying mute and unresponsive in his bathtub with an obvious severe burn of his right hand. Within several weeks, his condition improved but cognition and speech remained impaired. Subsequently, diabetes insipidus developed.

Examination

His stupor resolved over 1 week with treatment of bacteremia, but a profound global aphasia with some perseverative, nonfluent speech persisted. Initially, he had right arm and leg hemiplegia, with inability to move against gravity, and right hemineglect, but this resolved almost completely over 2 weeks. He was left with only a mild bilateral gait ataxia. Because of persistent and profound difficulties with expression and comprehension, nursing home placement was arranged.

Investigations

The initial drug screen was negative. Magnetic resonance imaging (MRI) demonstrated diffuse cortical signal abnormality and mild mass effect involving the cortex of much of the left cerebral hemisphere and cingulate cortex, with hypervascularity throughout the left cerebral hemisphere and cortical enhancement (Figure). Diffusion-weighted images demonstrated abnormal signal in the left cerebral hemisphere and cingulate gyrus. In addition, there were symmetric, minimally enhancing T_2-signal changes within the dorsal brainstem, extending from the posterolateral medulla through the dorsal pons, along the fourth ventricle, and into the cerebral peduncles, bilaterally. Radiographs of the long bones demonstrated medullary sclerosis. Computed tomography of the abdomen demonstrated a ring of soft tissue enveloping the aorta and kidneys. A diagnostic procedure was performed.

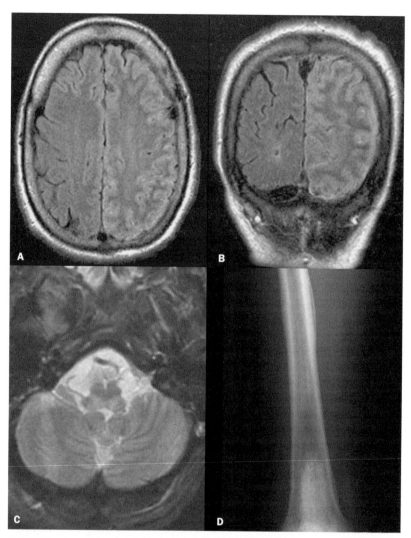

FIGURE. *A* and *B,* Axial and coronal MRI FLAIR images showing edema of the cerebral cortex of the left hemisphere. *C,* Axial T$_2$-weighted MRI showing symmetric T$_2$-signal changes in the dorsal brainstem. *D,* Radiograph of the femur demonstrating medullary sclerosis.

Commentary by Dr. David. F. Black

FHM is a rare, autosomal dominant form of migraine associated with episodic attacks of hemiplegia, aphasia, hemianopia, confusion, and sometimes coma, all of which may last several weeks and then resolve. If deficits persist, as in this case, a migrainous infarct is possible. Patients with FHM also have typical attacks of migraine with aura without hemiplegia.

FHM is associated with nine different mutations in the *CACNA1A* region of chromosome 19p13, and one of these can be found in approximately 50% of patients. Recently, mutations in the *ATP1A2* gene that encodes the α_2 subunit of the sodium-potassium pump linked to chromosome 1q23 have been found in families with FHM. The *CACNA1A* gene encodes for the α_{1A} subunit of a P/Q-type calcium channel that is expressed most densely in the cerebellum. Mutations of this gene are also associated with episodic ataxia type 2 and spinocerebellar ataxia type 6. According to anecdotal reports, intranasal ketamine, rapid intravenous administration of verapamil, or acetazolamide may have therapeutic benefit in acute attacks of FHM. Acetazolamide may also be useful prophylactically for FHM, although this has not been studied in a controlled fashion. Verapamil is often used prophylactically, yet the rationale for this is uncertain because verapamil inhibits the L-type rather than the P/Q-type calcium channel.

FHM can produce unilateral hemispheric changes seen on MRI, but the bilateral T_2-signal changes in the brainstem of our patient are not explained by migraine. The results of genetic screening for all known *CACNA1A* mutations in our patient were negative. ECD was suspected on clinical grounds because central diabetes insipidus, xanthelasmas, long-bone sclerosis, and retroperitoneal, mediastinal, and circumaortic fibrosis are typical for this disorder. Symmetric, bilateral long-bone medullary sclerosis is the most indicative—nearly a pathognomonic feature of ECD. The diagnosis was confirmed by examination of a femur biopsy specimen that showed non-Langerhans cell and foamy histiocytic infiltration.

ECD is a rare form of non-Langerhans histiocytosis, first described by William Chester and Jakob Erdheim in 1930. ECD may produce focal or diffuse histiocytic infiltration of almost any organ system, but the cause is unknown. No familial cases of ECD have been reported, to suggest a genetic cause. ECD is typically a progressive illness with variable severity. The most common neurologic sequelae include central diabetes insipidus and a slowly progressive cerebellar syndrome with gait ataxia. Our patient had nearly every reported symptom of ECD, although we do not know to what extent he had gait ataxia before his migrainous stroke. Severe forms of ECD are associated with decreased life span. Experimental therapies for ECD include corticosteroids, chemotherapy, and radiation, but thus far they have not proved to be notably efficacious.

The patient continues to have profound global aphasia and to reside in a nursing home. Occasionally, he is hospitalized for pulmonary infection or agitated behavior. In the future, his ECD may be treated with chemotherapy. Currently, he is not taking any preventive agent for migraine.

That two such rare diseases occurred simultaneously in the same person suggests a possible connection. Although other family members have hemiplegic migraine, to date none of them has symptoms of ECD.

REFERENCE

Wright RA, Hermann RC, Parisi JE. Neurological manifestations of Erdheim-Chester disease. *J Neurol Neurosurg Psychiatry* 1999;**66**:72-5.

History

A 5-year-old boy was born by induction after 40 weeks of gestation. Fetal movements, which began at 16 weeks, were feeble throughout gestation. Immediately after birth, he had a weak cry and suck, was hypotonic, and required intermittent respiratory support over the next 11 days. During the first year of life, he continued to have intermittent respiratory difficulties, some associated with apnea that required resuscitation. Eyelid ptosis was noted during infancy. At age 15 months, he underwent a fundoplication procedure for gastrointestinal reflux; tracheostomy and percutaneous gastrostomy were performed at the same time. He also had repeated episodes of pneumonia until the age of 3 years. Although he sat up at 7 months, he learned to walk only at 27 months but fell frequently. He fatigued easily. His speech became slurred and his eyes diverged when he was tired. The maternal great grandmother and one paternal cousin had droopy eyelids.

Examination

The patient had a pectus excavatum but no facial deformity. He walked with a slight waddle and footdrop. There was moderate to marked asymmetric eyelid ptosis and severe limitation of all ocular ductions but no diplopia (Figure). Manual muscle testing was unreliable but suggested moderate weakness of facial and proximal limb muscles and lesser weakness of the distal limb muscles. The tendon reflexes were hypoactive in the arms but normally active in the legs. Arm elevation time was limited to 20 seconds. The rest of the neurologic examination was unremarkable.

Investigations

Electromyographic studies revealed a defect of neuromuscular transmission. Stimulation of the facial and peroneal nerves at 2 Hz elicited a 10% decrement of the fifth compared with the first evoked compound muscle action potential (CMAP). The decremental response worsened following exercise and was improved by edrophonium and 3,4-diaminopyridine. Continuous 10-Hz stimulation of the peroneal nerve over 5 minutes decreased the initial CMAP amplitude by 80% to 90% and increased the decrement at 2 Hz to over 50%. Electrocardiography suggested right-axis deviation and right ventricular hypertrophy. The electroencephalogram was normal during wakefulness and sleep.

In vitro electrophysiologic studies of an intercostal muscle performed at rest and after conditioning trains of stimuli at 10 Hz for 5 minutes abolished the extracellularly recorded CMAP and the contractile response in less than 5 minutes. At the end of stimulation, the initial amplitude of the end plate potential (EPP) was decreased by 80% and the initial amplitude of the miniature EPP (MEPP), which was close to normal at rest, by 50%. (In normal subjects, a similar stimulation protocol decreases the EPP by less than 30% and does not significantly alter the MEPP amplitude.) Following stimulation, the observed electrophysiologic abnormalities disappeared slowly over 15 minutes. Patch-clamp studies of single acetylcholine receptor (AChR) channels showed that the conductance and kinetic properties of the AChR channel were normal. The number of AChRs per neuromuscular junction and the ultrastructure of the junction were normal.

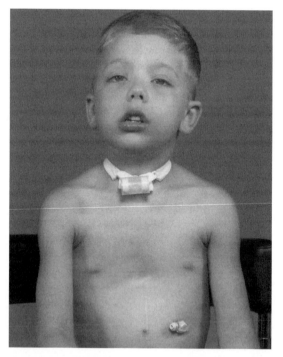

FIGURE. Patient at age 5. Note ptosis, esotropia, facial diplegia, tracheostomy, and percutaneous gastrostomy. (From Engel AG, Ohno K, Sine SM. In: Engel AG, Ed. *Myasthenia Gravis and Myasthenic Disorders.* New York: Oxford University Press; 1999:251-97. By permission of the publisher.)

Commentary by Dr. Andrew G. Engel

The clinical course and laboratory findings suggested a congenital myasthenic syndrome. The stimulation-dependent decrease of the MEPP amplitude in this patient was consistent with insufficient resynthesis or vesicular packaging of acetylcholine in response to increased functional demand. Candidate proteins for this type of defect are the presynaptic high-affinity choline transporter, ChAT, the vesicular acetylcholine transporter, and the vesicular proton pump. Direct sequencing of *CHAT* revealed two missense mutations in the *CHAT* coding region (R482G and R560H). Neither mutation had a significant effect on the level of ChAT protein expression in fibroblasts. However, analysis of the kinetic properties of the bacterially expressed and purified mutants showed that the R482G and R560H mutations reduced the catalytic efficiency of ChAT to 28% and 2% of wild type, respectively. The combined clinical, electromyographic, and laboratory findings established that the patient has a presynaptic congenital myasthenic syndrome caused by ChAT deficiency.

Congenital myasthenic syndromes are heterogeneous disorders caused by postsynaptic, synaptic, and presynaptic defects. Recent studies have identified congenital myasthenic syndromes caused by mutations in the postsynaptic AChR and in synaptic acetylcholinesterase, but the molecular basis of presynaptic congenital myasthenic syndrome has been elusive. The clinical features of the congenital myasthenic syndrome observed in our patient were first described in 1960 by Greer and Schotland. This syndrome presents at birth or in the neonatal period with hypotonia, variable eyelid ptosis, severe bulbar weakness causing dysphagia, and respiratory insufficiency with cyanosis and apnea. If the infant survives, the symptoms improve but the crises recur abruptly with infections, fever, excitement, vomiting, or overexertion. During crises, episodes of apnea can cause sudden death or anoxic brain injury. Between crises, patients may have only mild or no myasthenic symptoms. Because of the characteristic respiratory crises, we refer to this disease as "congenital myasthenic syndrome with episodic apnea." A similar phenotype could result from defects in the presynaptic high-affinity choline transporter, the vesicular acetylcholine transporter, or the vesicular proton pump, but no mutations of these proteins have been detected thus far in humans. Of note, a recently discovered congenital myasthenic syndrome caused by a mutation in the muscle sodium channel can also result in abrupt episodes of apnea.

An intriguing aspect of the ChAT deficiency syndrome is that none of the patients identified to date has central or autonomic nervous system symptoms. Currently, there is no evidence that tissue-specific isoforms explain the selective vulnerability of neuromuscular transmission. Reasons for this selective vulnerability may be owing to differences in presynaptic levels of ChAT, choline, or acetyl coenzyme A; rates of choline uptake; or rates of acetylcholine release under conditions of increased neuronal impulse flow. Although the reason for sparing of central and autonomic synapses is still not known, recognition of the syndrome is important because prophylactic anticholinesterase therapy can prevent or mitigate the attacks of respiratory distress, and prompt parenteral administration of a cholinesterase inhibitor at the onset of a crisis can be lifesaving.

REFERENCE

Ohno K, Tsujino A, Brengman JM, *et al.* Choline acetyltransferase mutations cause myasthenic syndrome associated with episodic apnea in humans. *Proc Natl Acad Sci USA* 2001;**98**:2017-22.

History

Two weeks after recovering from an episode of fever, vertigo, and vomiting, an 11-year-old boy was noted on a routine eye examination to have painless central loss of vision in the right eye. There was no recovery despite a course of treatment with intravenous and oral corticosteroids. Next, daily headache developed and was treated with doxycycline. The results of immunologic and serologic studies for Lyme disease, cat-scratch fever disease, and mycoplasma were normal. Acetazolamide was administered without noticeable benefit. The results of lumbar puncture were normal, but the opening pressure was recorded as 200 mm of H_2O. He had a past history of environmental allergies and repeated respiratory tract infections. The family history was unremarkable.

Examination

On examination, an ash-leaf spot was found on his abdomen and two small café-au-lait spots on his back. He had a right afferent pupillary defect. Acuity was reduced to 20/200 on the right. Visual field testing demonstrated a right central scotoma. Color vision was impaired in the right eye. Funduscopic examination showed optic disk edema and slight temporal pallor of the right optic nerve.

Investigations

The results of tests for vitamin B_{12}, tocopherol, free retinol, carboxyhemoglobin, cyanide, metals, homocysteine, and organic acids were normal. Findings on magnetic resonance imaging of the head were normal. The visual evoked response was absent on the right and prolonged on the left (123 ms; normal, <120 ms).

Commentary by Dr. Deborah L. Renaud

The differential diagnosis of optic neuropathy is broad. Ischemic vascular forms of optic neuropathy are more common in older patients. Pain generally accompanies the visual loss in cases of inflammatory optic neuritis. Compressive or infiltrative lesions that affect the optic nerve, such as optic glioma or optic nerve sheath meningioma, may present with painless unilateral visual loss. Neoplastic and non-neoplastic causes of compression of the intracranial optic nerve and optic chiasm frequently present with visual field defects. Slowly progressive, symmetric, central visual loss suggests a possible toxic or nutritional cause. Hereditary optic neuropathies generally are classified by their mode of inheritance: autosomal dominant, autosomal recessive, or mitochondrial (maternal) inheritance. Symptoms may be confined to the visual system or be accompanied by other neurologic or systemic signs and symptoms. Optic neuropathy can also be a manifestation of inherited metabolic and degenerative diseases.

Historical clues are often essential to determining the cause of optic neuropathy. The temporal sequence of visual symptoms, the presence or absence of pain, the family history, and associated neurologic signs and symptoms are important elements of the history. In this case, the history of unilateral painless central visual loss in an otherwise healthy young boy is suggestive of a hereditary optic neuropathy. Mitochondrial DNA analysis demonstrated a mutation at position 11,778 consistent with a diagnosis of Leber's hereditary optic neuropathy.

Leber's hereditary optic neuropathy (Online Mendelian Inheritance in Man [OMIM] 535000) is maternally inherited. The incidence is approximately 1 in 25,000 to 1 in 50,000 worldwide. Males are predominantly affected, with a male-to-female ratio of approximately 4:1. The usual age at onset of symptoms is 15 to 35 years, but onset can occur anytime from the first to the seventh decade. Patients present with painless central visual loss and early impairment of color vision. Most commonly, the visual loss is initially monocular, with involvement of the second eye weeks to months later. The degree of visual impairment is variable, but frequently visual acuity is 20/200 or less. Up to 60% of patients have some improvement in visual acuity later in the course. During the acute phase, ophthalmoscopy may show a circumpapillary telangiectatic microangiopathy and swelling of the retinal nerve fiber layer (Figure) or the findings may be normal. Optic atrophy eventually develops. The majority of patients with Leber's hereditary optic neuropathy are otherwise healthy, although cardiac conduction abnormalities, movement disorders, neuropathy, and multiple sclerosis-like features have been described in a small subset of patients. So far, treatment has failed to prevent or reverse the visual loss in patients with this optic neuropathy. Three primary mitochondrial DNA point mutations, G3460A, G11778A, and T14484C, account for approximately 85% to 95% of the pathogenic mutations in patients with Leber's hereditary optic neuropathy. These genes encode subunits of complex I of the mitochondrial respiratory chain. Incomplete penetrance has been noted in families with this condition, with expression of the phenotype in only 50% of males and 10% of females carrying the pathogenic mutation. An interaction between mitochondrial and nuclear genetic influences as well as environmental factors may account for this variability in penetrance. Heteroplasmy of mitochondrial DNA may also contribute. Genetic counseling is recommended.

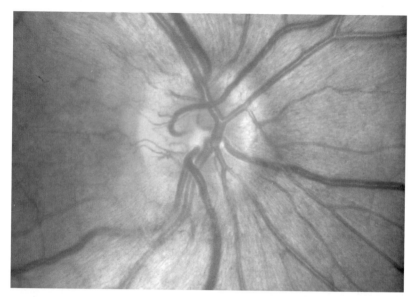

FIGURE. Fundus photograph demonstrating typical circumpapillary telangiectatic microangiopathy and swelling of the retinal nerve fiber layer (see color insert).

REFERENCE

Man PY, Turnbull DM, Chinnery PF. Leber hereditary optic neuropathy. *J Med Genet* 2002;**39**:162-9.

History

A 72-year-old woman first noted problems with leg strength at age 40. She needed to use her arms to arise from a chair, had progressive trouble climbing steps, fell frequently, and described a waddling gait. With a 10-year history of progressive dysphagia for solids, she gradually lost 25 lb. Removal of tori from her oropharynx 5 years previously (at age 67) was unhelpful. Her speech had worsened, becoming soft and "cracking." She had difficulty articulating "C" and "G" and drooled at night. The family history was noncontributory.

Examination

Her voice was high-pitched, dysprosodic, and indistinct for labial consonants. The tongue was weak, without fasciculations. She had atrophy of the shoulder girdle and thighs, without fasciculations or myotonia. There was symmetrical weakness in a limb-girdle distribution, with hip flexors and adductors affected most severely. The intrinsic hand muscles were weak. Deep tendon reflexes were absent. The sensory examination was normal. The gait was hip-waddling, with hyperextension of the knees.

Investigations

The results of routine biochemistry and hematology studies were normal. Creatine kinase and thyroid-stimulating hormone levels were normal; the serum aldolase level was mildly elevated. Serum protein electrophoresis demonstrated a 0.5-g/dL IgG λ monoclonal protein. A skeletal bone survey was negative. A video swallow examination showed severe oropharyngeal dysphagia, decreased peristalsis, and abnormal epiglottic excursion. The forced vital capacity was 42%, and the maximal inspiratory pressure was decreased to 23% of the predicted value. Overnight oximetry documented nocturnal desaturation (<90%) for 3% of the recording time. Nerve conduction studies were normal apart from the absence of phrenic responses. Electromyography (EMG) demonstrated fibrillation potentials, myotonic discharges, and small complex motor unit potentials in the paraspinal muscles and the left diaphragm but no abnormalities in limb muscles. A diagnostic deltoid muscle biopsy was performed, followed shortly by the development of intermittent atrial flutter and atrial fibrillation.

Commentary by Dr. E. Peter Bosch

Type II glycogenosis (glycogen storage disease [GSD-II]) is an autosomal recessive lysosomal storage disorder caused by partial or complete deficiency of acid α-glucosidase activity (GAA), or acid maltase. This enzyme defect results in the accumulation of lysosomal glycogen in many tissues, with cardiac and skeletal muscle affected most severely (Figure). The estimated prevalence of GSD-II is low (1 in 40,000 to 100,000 newborns).

Three forms of the disease have been recognized. The infantile form (or Pompe's disease) results from complete or near complete deficiency of GAA and presents within the first 3 months of life with hypotonia, progressive weakness, macroglossia, hypertrophic cardiomyopathy, and hepatomegaly. Its course is invariably fatal, and the child dies of cardiorespiratory failure before age 2 years. The juvenile form presents in the first decade with proximal weakness and mild or no cardiac involvement and leads to respiratory failure in the second or third decade of life. The adult-onset form begins in the third to seventh decade (range, 18-65 years). Most patients present with pelvic girdle weakness affecting predominantly the gluteal muscles and thigh adductors, followed by proximal arm weakness. Trunk extensors and abdominal muscles are frequently affected. Up to 30% of patients present with respiratory dysfunction. Orthopnea, frequent nocturnal arousals, morning headaches, and excessive daytime drowsiness suggest nocturnal hypoventilation and early respiratory insufficiency. Diaphragmatic weakness is found in 58% of patients at initial evaluation. Face or tongue weakness occurs in 13% of patients, but macroglossia is rare. Cardiac enlargement is not found in the adult form. Respiratory failure is the main cause of death. The disease is often misdiagnosed as polymyositis or limb-girdle muscular dystrophy, as it was in our patient. Clues leading to the correct diagnosis include selective involvement of respiratory and truncal muscles and myotonic discharges on needle EMG.

Serum creatine kinase levels are increased (1.5-10 times normal) in 95% of patients. Needle EMG findings are abnormal in 94% of patients, with small-amplitude, short-duration myopathic motor units and early recruitment. More specifically, needle insertion induces myotonic discharges. Myotonic potentials are especially prominent in the paraspinal muscles in 30% of patients.

Electrocardiographic abnormalities are mild and nonspecific. Respiratory muscle involvement should be investigated by measuring forced vital capacity with the patient upright and supine and maximal respiratory pressures and performing overnight oximetry. Muscle biopsy specimens demonstrate a vacuolar myopathy. In the adult form, vacuoles are present in 25% to 75% of fibers but may be absent in unaffected muscles. The vacuoles react strongly with the periodic acid–Schiff stain. The vacuoles also react with acid phosphatase, confirming that they are secondary lysosomes. Although the enzyme defect can be detected in leukocytes and skin fibroblasts, biochemical analysis of GAA in muscle tissue establishes the diagnosis.

The human *GAA* gene has been mapped to the long arm of chromosome 17 (17q25.2-q25.3); it contains 20 exons and has a length of 28 kb. To date, more than 70 mutations have been identified. Missense and nonsense mutations, splicing defects, deletions, and insertions have been described. Most patients are compound heterozygotes of the *GAA* gene. There is usually an inverse relation between residual enzyme activity and clinical severity. The most common mutant allele in the adult-onset variant is a 13 T to G splice site mutation in intron 1.

Treatment is still mainly supportive. Noninvasive positive pressure ventilation is instituted for nocturnal hypoventilation or daytime respiratory failure. Our patient was given anticoagulant therapy with warfarin (atrial fibrillation), started receiving noninvasive positive pressure ventilation at night, and was instructed to consume a high protein, low carbohydrate diet. Dietary treatment with a high protein diet has produced contradictory results. Intravenous enzyme replacement therapy using recombinant human GAA purified from transgenic rabbit milk has shown promising results in open-label clinical trials of patients with infantile disease. All treated patients survived beyond 1 year with normal cardiac function. Gene therapy is being actively investigated in both in vitro and animal models.

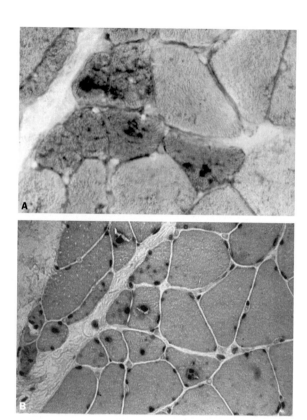

FIGURE. *A,* Deltoid muscle biopsy specimen. Several fibers contain focally increased glycogen. (Periodic acid–Schiff; original magnification, x160.) *B,* Many muscle fibers contain multiple acid phosphatase-positive vacuoles and granules. (Acid phosphatase; original magnification, x100.) Acid maltase deficiency was confirmed by in vitro biochemical studies (8.4% of normal values, 63-123 μM/[min · g tissue]) (see color insert). (Courtesy of Dr. A. E. Engel.)

REFERENCE

Raben N, Plotz P, Byrne BJ. Acid α-glucosidase deficiency (glycogenosis type II, Pompe disease). *Curr Mol Med* 2002;**2**:145-66.

History

For several years, a 78-year-old woman was aware that she lost consciousness when lying supine or sitting up straight in a car. Sitting sideways in a car and avoiding lying on her back prevented the recurrence of these episodes. On several occasions, she had lost consciousness when she bumped her low back climbing into a car. The episodes were quickly terminated if she could be lifted to an upright posture. Many episodes were followed by headache. While she was unconscious, her appearance was described as "flushed" or "normal color." Occasionally, she noted a deep pressure discomfort in her low back while standing in one position. She experienced a 15-minute period of "unresponsiveness" during a carotid ultrasonographic study in the supine posture at a "vascular disease screening center" before her evaluation at Mayo Clinic. Upon resuming an upright posture, she remained confused for several minutes and complained of headache and severe unilateral visual loss (later attributed to bilateral, asymmetric intraretinal hemorrhages).

She had a history of a fall that led to low back pain at age 20 years. Radiographs showed "spina bifida." Her low back pain improved but never resolved. At age 53, she fell again, but there was major change in the low back pain. Thereafter, an enlarging lump was noted in the lower end of the spine. Several years later, aspiration of the mass revealed crystal clear cerebrospinal fluid (CSF).

Examination

Physical examination demonstrated pes cavus with hammertoe deformities and absence of ankle jerks. A fluctuant 12-cm mass was noted overlying the mid-sacrum just lateral to the midline.

Investigations

Spine magnetic resonance imaging (MRI) demonstrated a large, multilobulated, communicating sacral meningocele and tethered cord (Figure). Brain MRI showed atrophy only.

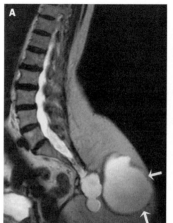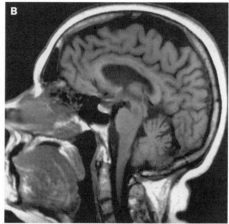

FIGURE. *A,* Sagittal T$_2$-weighted magnetic resonance image of the spine distal to the low thoracic level shows a large multilobulated communicating meningocele, with its largest component between the coccyx and skin. It is evident how pressure from the posterior aspect (*arrows*) can lead to displacement of cerebrospinal fluid from the meningocele sac into the spinal thecal sac. (From Bekavac I, Halloran JI. *AJNR Am J Neuroradiol* 2003;**24**:838-9. By permission of the American Society of Neuroradiology.) *B,* Right sagittal T$_1$-weighted magnetic resonance image of the brain shows only atrophy but no Chiari malformation.

Commentary by Dr. Bahram Mokri

In adults, a posterior lumbosacral meningocele is typically a posttrau-
matic or postsurgical development. They rarely occur spontaneously.
They are meningeal herniations through defects in the posterior vertebral compartments that may or may not contain neural elements. They
can be small or large and symptomatic or asymptomatic. Additional
anatomic or pathologic abnormalities may sometimes be associated
with lumbosacral meningoceles. The patient reported here had a large
posterior sacral meningocele, likely traumatic in origin, and an asymptomatic, associated tethered cord. The stereotypical mode of provoca-
tion of symptoms (lying supine, leaning back with pressure against the
dorsal lumbosacral area) strongly suggests that the symptoms were
related directly to quick displacement of CSF from the meningocele sac
into the thecal sac, with a subsequent increase in intracranial pressure.
This would lead to a secondary increase in cerebral venous pressure,
which in turn could result in decreased cerebral blood flow. Decreased
cerebral blood flow would explain the episodes of loss of consciousness. Increased cerebral venous pressure was likely responsible for
the retinal hemorrhages. In the early decades of the 19th century, the
French physiologist Magendie convinced his contemporaries of com-
munication between the fluids that filled the cranial and spinal
spaces, thus the term "cerebrospinal fluid." Among several observa-
tions made by Magendie was that pressure on meningoceles in infants
with open fontanelles caused the fontanelles to bulge. According to the
Monro-Kellie hypothesis, with an intact and noncompressible skull, as
in normal adults, an increase in CSF volume should cause a decrease in
intracranial blood volume because the brain volume remains relatively
constant. In the patient reported here, pressure on the meningocele
likely caused displacement of only a fraction of the CSF in the sac.
Because this was an acute displacement, it was apparently enough to

cause a symptomatic increase in intracranial pressure. Acute displacement of a given volume of CSF can lead to more than a casually expected increase in CSF pressure because with an intact skull the relation between CSF volume and pressure is exponential rather than linear. It has been shown experimentally that uniform increments in CSF volume cause progressively larger increases in CSF pressure.

REFERENCE

Miller JD. Volume and pressure in the craniospinal axis. *Clin Neurosurg* 1975;**22**:76-105.

History

A 66-year-old man had a 2-year history of back and right buttock pain aggravated by standing. Epidural corticosteroid injections provided some benefit. In the subsequent months, subacute, painless, progressive symmetrical weakness of the lower limbs (proximal greater than distal) developed, making it difficult for him to arise from a chair. He fell repeatedly. He had no bowel, bladder, or sensory complaints. The possibility of statin-induced myopathy was considered, but his symptoms persisted despite discontinuation of these agents (the serum level of creatine kinase was normal). Electromyography (EMG) and muscle and nerve biopsies were performed at a tertiary referral center. The muscle biopsy specimen was interpreted as normal. However, on the basis of slowed nerve conduction velocities and "collections of inflammatory cells" seen in the sural nerve biopsy specimen, corticosteroid therapy was started for the presumed diagnosis of chronic inflammatory poly-radiculopathy. There was partial improvement in his leg weakness. He had a past medical history of smoking, type 2 diabetes mellitus, hyperlipidemia, and aortoiliac bypass surgery. He came to Mayo Clinic for a second opinion. When asked, he stated that he had a dry mouth and was impotent.

Examination

Neurologic examination demonstrated symmetrical weakness of the lower extremity, proximal greater than distal. Sensory examination findings were normal. The deep tendon reflexes were reduced but preserved. His gait suggested marked proximal muscle weakness.

Investigations

The erythrocyte sedimentation rate was elevated at 58 mm/h (normal, <22 mm/h). Nerve conduction studies and EMG were performed, followed by additional studies.

Commentary by Dr. C. Michel Harper, Jr.

Nerve conduction studies demonstrated low-amplitude compound muscle action potentials (CMAPs) with slowed conduction velocities, consistent with a peripheral neuropathy. Because the patient had proximal weakness, dry mouth, impotence, and a history of smoking, repetitive stimulation studies were performed (Figure). Repetitive stimulation of the ulnar, peroneal, and spinal accessory nerves demonstrated a 57% decrement of the ulnar CMAP, a 33% decrement of the spinal accessory CMAP, and a 40% decrement of the peroneal CMAP. The ulnar CMAP amplitude demonstrated 300% facilitation (3-fold increase) after 10 seconds of exercise. Less prominent facilitation was noted in the spinal accessory and peroneal CMAPs. Needle examination demonstrated small, polyphasic varying motor unit potentials in most muscles studied. The electrodiagnostic findings were those of a presynaptic defect of neuromuscular transmission consistent with the diagnosis of LEMS. The diagnosis was confirmed when serum levels of P/Q voltage-gated calcium channel (VGCC) antibodies were elevated to 2,094 pmol/L (normal, <20 pmol/L). Computed tomography of the chest showed a 2-cm mass at the left hilum, subsequently demonstrated on transbronchial biopsy to be SCLC.

The patient experienced little benefit when treated with pyridostigmine but improved after symptomatic treatment with 3,4-diaminopyridine, which enhances the release of acetylcholine (ACh) from the motor nerve terminal. Chemotherapy and prophylactic whole-brain radiotherapy led to remission of the SCLC, followed by gradual improvement in the manifestations of LEMS.

LEMS is an autoimmune presynaptic disorder of neuromuscular transmission characterized by proximal fatigable weakness, reduced tendon reflexes, and mild autonomic dysfunction (e.g., dry mouth, impotence). The clinical and electrophysiologic features of LEMS, including its association with SCLC, were first described by Lambert, Eaton, and Rooke in 1956. Subsequent microelectrode studies established LEMS as a presynaptic disorder by demonstrating a decrease in the size of the end plate potential and reduced quantal release of ACh.

The P/Q VGCC, which controls calcium influx and ACh release from the nerve terminal, is the presumptive antigenic target of autoantibodies that mediate LEMS. Several lines of evidence support an autoimmune origin of LEMS. First, serologic tests for P/Q VGCC antibodies are positive in 90% of patients with LEMS. Second, P/Q VGCCs are expressed by SCLC, a neoplasm observed in 60% of cases of LEMS. Third, LEMS typically improves with successful treatment of SCLC. Fourth, the presynaptic defect of neuromuscular transmission characteristic of LEMS can be passively transferred to mice with IgG from LEMS patients. Finally, immunomodulating therapy (e.g., plasmapheresis, intravenous immunoglobulin, corticosteroids) is effective in the treatment of LEMS.

LEMS is a rare disorder, and a high index of clinical suspicion is needed to make the diagnosis, particularly when other diseases (e.g., peripheral neuropathy) are present. Fatigable muscle weakness of the proximal hip girdle, dryness of the mouth, impotence, and a strong smoking history are important clues that should lead to serologic tests for VGCC antibodies or to EMG. The electromyographer should always check for facilitation even if there is evidence for a peripheral neuropathy in the appropriate clinical setting. Areflexia is often listed as a cardinal feature of LEMS, but as this case illustrates, reflexes sometimes are preserved in LEMS. If reflexes are reduced, facilitation of the reflex after 10 seconds of exercise is a useful bedside test for LEMS and is easier to detect than facilitation of muscle strength.

Findings of "nonspecific" inflammation in a sural nerve or muscle biopsy specimen can be misleading and do not always confirm the diagnosis of chronic inflammatory demyelinating polyradiculoneuropathy or inflammatory myopathy.

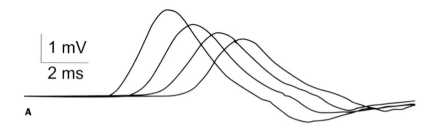

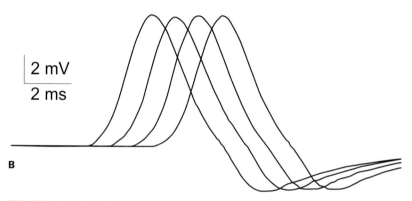

FIGURE. Results of repetitive stimulation of the ulnar nerve before (*A*) and immediately after (*B*) 10 seconds of isometric exercise. The ulnar nerve was stimulated at the wrist at 2 Hz, and the recording was made over the abductor digiti minimi muscle. The ulnar compound muscle action potential demonstrates 300% facilitation (3-fold increase) after exercise, consistent with a presynaptic defect of neuromuscular transmission.

REFERENCE

Harper CM, Lennon VA. Lambert-Eaton syndrome: dedicated to Dr. Edward H. Lambert on the occasion of his 87th birthday. In: Kaminski HJ, Ed. *Myasthenia Gravis and Related Disorders*. Totowa, NJ: Humana Press; 2003:269-91.

History

A 68-year-old woman who smoked for 42 years developed bilateral subscapular, steady aching pain that radiated to both upper extremities along the ulnar aspects to the hands and numbness in the ulnar three fingers bilaterally. She then noticed the gradual onset of weakness in the legs and numbness in the toes. Her balance deteriorated such that she had difficulty walking and used a cane.

Three months after the onset of these symptoms, vision became blurry in both eyes, but worse on the right, especially in the lower field. She noticed floaters. She lost 20 lb over 4 months and suffered bloating after meals. There was a history of chronic diarrhea, but this had not changed. The patient said she did not have bladder symptoms, changes in sweating, or light-headedness. She expressed no concern about her intellectual functioning.

Examination

Mental status was normal. Visual acuity was 20/70 OD and 20/20 OS. Visual field testing showed peripheral constriction bilaterally and, in addition, an inferior altitudinal defect on the right. The patient read 10/10 color plates OU. The right optic disk was swollen, and the left one was normal (Figure). There were rare small nonclumped cells in the posterior vitreous in both eyes. There was no pars planitis. The rest of the cranial nerves were normal.

Both legs were weak. The patient was unable to get out of a chair without using her arms to push herself up. Distal strength was better. The patient was able to stand on heels and toes. Sensory testing demonstrated loss to pinprick in the ulnar forearms and hands. There was also mild distal loss in the lower extremities. The deep tendon reflexes were normal, with no pathologic reflexes. There was no appendicular ataxia, but the gait was very wide-based and ataxic. The patient needed the support of another person to walk.

Investigations

The erythrocyte sedimentation rate was 44 mm/h. Electromyography showed mild bilateral C8-T1 radiculopathies. Paraspinal fibrillations and larger motor units in some lower extremity muscles suggested involvement of anterior horn cells or their roots at multiple thoracic and upper lumbar levels. Electroretinographic abnormalities included prolongation of the scotopic combined rod-cone (maximal) responses, the photopic cone response, the scotopic rod response, and the photopic 30-Hz flicker response. Computed tomography of the chest showed a mass in the lung, with mediastinal involvement. Bronchoscopic findings were unremarkable. Additional diagnostic studies were performed.

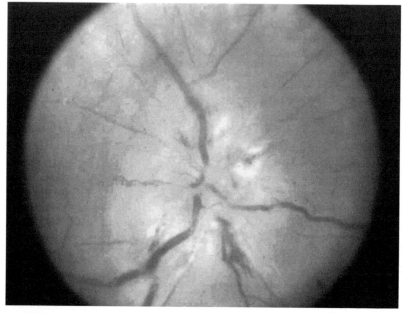

FIGURE. Fundus photograph demonstrating optic disk swelling with hemorrhages (see color insert).

DIAGNOSIS CASE 46

Paraneoplastic optic neuritis, polyradiculopathy, and ataxia for which collapsin response mediator protein-5 (CRMP-5) autoantibody serves as a serologic marker

Commentary by Dr. Shelley A. Cross

Paraneoplastic antibody screening showed CRMP-5 autoantibody at a titer of 1/3,840. The glutamic acid decarboxylase (GAD)65 antibody was also positive. The carcinoma-associated retinopathy antibody was negative. Lumbar puncture was not performed. Mediastinoscopy with biopsy revealed small cell lung cancer.

This case represents a paraneoplastic subacute encephalomyelo-radiculoneuropathy with optic neuritis accompanied by vitreous inflammatory cells (and sometimes by retinitis and intrathecal inflammatory cells) associated with small cell carcinoma. CRMP-5 is its serologic marker. Although CRMP-5-IgG is a marker of autoimmunity initiated by either small cell carcinoma or thymoma, we have not encountered a patient with optic neuritis, retinitis, and thymoma. Cases similar to the one presented here have been reported since 1986, but only recently has the syndrome been fully described, the antibody clearly identified, and the ophthalmologic and neurologic features described in detail.

Patients may present with subacute visual loss, swollen optic disks, vascular sheathing in the retina, and cells in the posterior vitreous. This presentation can be mistaken for ocular lymphoma and has led to vitreous biopsy.

Common neurologic accompaniments to visual symptoms include other cranial neuropathies (particularly loss of taste and smell) and subacute chorea or other basal ganglia disorders. However, a much larger variety of abnormalities can be seen. Mental status abnormalities can include dementia, cognitive slowing, and partial complex seizures. Cranial nerve abnormalities include cranial mononeuropathies (including bulbar and retrobulbar optic neuritis) and ocular motility disorders that reflect brainstem dysfunction.

Motor and sensory findings reflect involvement of both the central and peripheral nervous systems: polyradiculoneuropathy, mononeuropathy, peripheral neuropathy, unspecified muscle weakness, Lambert-Eaton syndrome, and myelopathy. Movement disorders include parkinsonism, chorea, hemiballismus, dyskinesias, and akathesia. Cerebellar manifestations include ataxia and nystagmus. Autonomic abnormalities are common and include orthostatic intolerance, nausea, early satiety, constipation or diarrhea, dry mouth, and weight loss greater than 20 lb attributed partly to gastrointestinal dysautonomia. The presentation of a few patients superficially resembles that of Devic's disease (neuromyelitis optica).

The progression of the disease is subacute, and the symptoms and findings can wax and wane. Magnetic resonance imaging demonstrates patchy T_2-signal changes that sometimes show enhancement. CRMP-5-IgG is detected in the serum and frequently in the cerebrospinal fluid (CSF). Pleocytosis, increased protein concentration, increased IgG synthesis, and oligoclonal bands are found on CSF analysis. There may be pleocytosis in the vitreous. Cytologic study of the CSF and vitreous biopsy specimen shows reactive cells, mostly CD8+ cells without the large size, clumping, and monoclonal origin characteristic of lymphoma cells.

Pathologically, this entity is one of inflammatory infiltrates composed of T cells, mostly CD8+ cells. There is prominent perivascular cuffing and patchy loss of axons and myelin. CRMP-5 immunoreactivity has been identified in both the optic nerve and retina. This observation supports the hypothesis that the pertinent immunogen inducing the clinical features of this disorder is a tumor-derived CRMP-5 peptide. This peptide is a surrogate marker for cytotoxic T-cell activation.

Recognition of this entity is important because it expedites the search for malignancy. Lung neoplasms associated with CRMP-5-IgG are the small cell type in at least 77% of cases, are generally limited in spread, and can be difficult to find. If computed tomographic findings in the chest are negative, positron emission tomography may be useful. The possibility of an extrapulmonary primary source should be considered. Identification of the CRMP-5-IgG antibody will obviate the need for vitreous biopsy.

Treatment is experimental and focuses on the underlying malignancy and immunosuppression.

REFERENCE

Cross SA, Salomao DR, Parisi JE, *et al*. Paraneoplastic autoimmune optic neuritis with retinitis defined by CRMP-5-IgG. *Ann Neurol* 2003;**54**:38-50.

History

A 49-year-old man had a 4-week episode of severe right temporal head-ache and diplopia 13 years ago that resolved spontaneously. One year later, he had a 4-week episode of left-hand weakness and diplopia. He reported a 12-year history of slowly progressive leg weakness with gait instability, a 9-year history of reduced short-term memory, and an 8-year history of mild arm weakness. Multiple sclerosis was diagnosed after a cerebrospinal fluid (CSF) study showed increased synthesis of IgG. Eight years ago, he had a 4-week episode of gait imbalance, nausea, and vomiting that resolved with intravenous corticosteroid treatment. Six years ago, he noted reduced peripheral vision, paresthesias of the feet, and episodic leg spasms. Four years ago, treatment with interferon β-1b injections was started. Two years ago, constipation, bladder urgency, frequency, double voiding, and incontinence developed. His memory worsened.

Fourteen months before his evaluation, he experienced a 20-minute aphasic episode, followed 2 hours later by a fall to the floor without loss of consciousness and incoherent speech. Angiography showed a focal 50% stenosis of the left vertebral artery at the skull base near the origin of the posterior inferior cerebellar artery. For 15 months, he received treatment daily with cyclophosphamide, combined with occasional oral steroid pulses lasting from days to several weeks. His past medical history also included recurrent inguinal and abdominal lymphadenopathy diagnosed intraoperatively at ages 23 and 27. He required a cane to walk following hip replacement for a traumatic fracture at age 33. Five years ago, he developed a dry cough with increasing dyspnea on exertion, and treatment was started with montelukast (Singulair) and a combination of fluticasone and salmeterol (Advair) for presumed asthma. He had inflammatory polyarthritis with a positive rheumatoid factor on one occasion 8 years ago, herpes zoster 6 years ago, and a recent pulmonary embolism. He had not been exposed to human immunodeficiency virus or tuberculosis. His paternal aunt had multiple sclerosis.

Examination

On neurologic examination, eye movements were ataxic and saccadic and mild to moderate upper motor neuron weakness involved all four limbs, more so in the right proximal leg and left distal L5/S1-innervated muscles. Hyperreflexia was present, although both brachial radialis and left ankle reflexes were diminished. The right leg was slightly spastic. The Babinski response was elicited bilaterally. A stocking sensory loss to pinprick was demonstrated on the sensory examination, and vibration sense was diminished at the toes. Gait was antalgic and spastic, with the right leg circumducting more than the left leg.

Investigations

Laboratory tests demonstrated a mild macrocytic anemia of 10.1 g (mean corpuscular volume, 101 fL; normal, 81.2-95.1 fL). The erythrocyte sedimentation rate was elevated at 43 mm/h (normal, <22 mm/h). Alkaline phosphatase was increased at 528 U/L (normal, 98-251 U/L) entirely from the bone fraction. Serum levels of angiotensin-converting enzyme and calcium were both normal. Hypogammaglobulinemia was detected. The CSF was acellular. CSF protein was elevated to twice the normal value, although the IgG level was normal. The cell count and cytologic features were normal, and one oligoclonal band was present (normal). Chest radiography disclosed mild nodularity in both lungs, with discrete nodules in the right base and right upper lung, and a mild prominence of the right hilum. Computed tomography of the spine demonstrated sclerosis of vertebral bodies L1, L2, and L5. Electromyography demonstrated an old left C7 radiculopathy, a mild right S1 radiculopathy, and a chronic, active left L5 radiculopathy with no evidence of peripheral neuropathy. Tibial somatosensory evoked potentials (SSEPs) were abnormal, but median SSEPs and visual evoked responses were normal.

Magnetic resonance imaging (MRI) demonstrated periventricular lesions prominently involving the centrum semiovale of both cerebral hemispheres, with extension to involve fibers of the corpus callosum (Figure). Several small lesions were present in the superior cerebellar peduncles bilaterally. A focal wedge-shaped area of increased signal intensity in the posteromedial aspect of the left cerebellar hemisphere was associated with prominent leptomeningeal enhancement involving the medial aspect of both occipital lobes in the vicinity of the calcarine cortices and within the superior vermis. Subtle leptomeningeal enhancement involved the inferior left frontal lobe. MRI of the lumbar spine, with and without contrast, demonstrated multiple low-signal intensity enhancing masses within the vertebral bodies. Mild smooth leptomeningeal nerve root enhancement was noted within the cauda equina as well as enlargement of the left S1 nerve root.

A diagnostic study was performed.

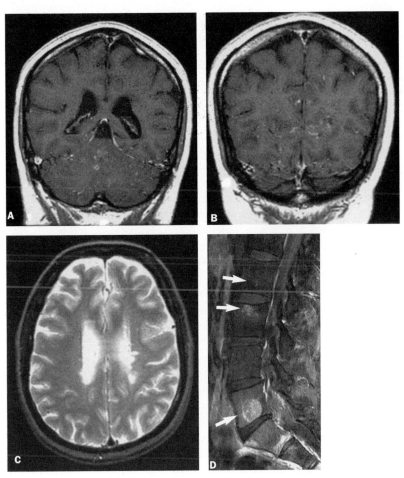

FIGURE. Contrast and noncontrast MRIs of the brain and lumbar spine. *A* and *B*, Coronal postcontrast image of the brain shows prominent leptomeningeal enhancement involving the medial aspect of both occipital lobes in the vicinity of the calcarine cortices and within the superior vermis. *C*, A T_2-weighted image shows multiple periventricular white matter lesions indistinguishable from those of multiple sclerosis. *D*, A contrast study of the lumbar spine demonstrates multiple low-signal intensity enhancing masses within the vertebral bodies (*arrows*). The largest mass, in vertebral body L5, is approximately 2 cm in diameter.

Commentary by Dr. Claudia F. Lucchinetti

Sarcoidosis is a multisystem granulomatous disease of unknown cause characterized pathologically by the presence of noncaseating granulomas, particularly in the lung and lymph nodes (but they can occur in any organ system). It most commonly affects persons 20 to 40 years old and is often associated with the development of chronic progressive disease in patients older than 40 years. The disease incidence is highest in U.S. black and Scandinavian populations and is less common among U.S. white, Japanese, Indian, Spanish, and South American populations. The disease is thought to result from a complex interaction of multiple genes with environmental exposures or infection.

Patients with sarcoidosis may be entirely asymptomatic or have a wide range of constitutional and other nonspecific symptoms, including respiratory complaints (dry cough, dyspnea, chest pain), skin rashes (erythema nodosum, papules, nodules, plaques), systemic symptoms (fever, night sweats, fatigue, malaise), ocular symptoms (pain, visual change), and musculoskeletal symptoms (joint pains, myalgias).

Approximately 90% of patients with sarcoidosis have pulmonary involvement, with either bilateral hilar adenopathy or interstitial disease. Patients often mistakenly receive treatment for a more common pulmonary disease such as bronchitis or asthma. The lymph nodes, eyes, bone marrow, spleen, liver, kidneys, salivary glands, skin, and mucous membranes are all potential sites of involvement. Osseous sarcoidosis occurs in 1% to 13% of patients, usually in the setting of chronic sarcoidosis. When present, it is usually in the bone marrow of the phalangeal bones of the hands and feet; however, it also has been noted less frequently in the marrow space of the long bones of the extremities, ribs, vertebral bodies, and calvarium. The lesions can be lytic and destructive.

In approximately 5% of the patients, the central nervous system (CNS) is involved, although postmortem studies have suggested that antemortem diagnosis is made in only 50% of these patients. Nervous system involvement may be the presenting feature in more than one-third of the patients, and virtually any part of the neuraxis can be involved. In some patients, the disease may remain restricted to the nervous system. Susceptible sites include the cranial nerves (optic>facial>glossopharyngeal>vagus>cochlear), meninges, hypothalamus, pituitary gland, spinal cord, peripheral nerves, and muscle. Spinal cord syndromes range from intramedullary tumorlike presentations to meningitic-radicular syndromes.

The wide spectrum of clinical presentations makes sarcoidosis a diagnostic and therapeutic challenge. Because of the clinical overlap with Wegener's granulomatosis, lymphoma, carcinoma, fungal disease, and mycobacterial infections, additional testing is needed to exclude these possibilities. An occupational and environmental exposure history should be obtained and a tuberculin skin test performed. Serum angiotensin-converting enzyme levels do not reliably correlate with disease activity or response to treatment. Often, the investigation to establish the diagnosis focuses on searching for histologic confirmation in other organs. A complete neurologic examination, electrocardiography, and complete ophthalmologic examination are needed to exclude the involvement of critical organs. To determine the extent and severity of disease, the following are indicated: chest radiography, pulmonary function testing, liver enzyme measurements, renal assessment (electrolytes, blood urea nitrogen, creatinine levels), urinalysis, complete blood count, and serum calcium levels.

In cases of neurosarcoidosis, biopsy of CNS tissue may be required to make a definitive diagnosis. When investigating for neurosarcoidosis, a full neurophthalmologic work-up is indicated, including a search for both anterior and posterior segment disease with a slit-lamp examination and fluorescein angiography as well as conjunctival biopsies. CSF abnormalities are common in neurosarcoidosis and most often include an increased protein concentration and CSF lymphocytosis with occasional rare neutrophils and monocytes. Oligoclonal bands and an increased CSF IgG index and synthesis rate may be present. The range of abnormalities seen on MRI includes white matter lesions, hydrocephalus, mass lesions in brain parenchyma, meningeal enhancement, enhancement of parenchymal lesions, and lesions of the optic nerves and spinal cord, with or without enlargement of these structures. Occasionally, white matter lesions seen in neurosarcoidosis are indistinguishable from those of multiple sclerosis, as in our patient. Although none of the MRI appearances is specific for neurosarcoidosis, meningeal enhancement or persistent enhancement (beyond 6 weeks) is more suggestive of a granulomatous process and is not expected in multiple sclerosis.

The symptoms and clinical findings of sarcoidosis tend to wax and wane spontaneously or in response to therapy. Spontaneous, complete clinical remissions with resolution of abnormal radiographic findings occur in a notable number of patients who do not receive treatment. Approximately one-third of patients with neurosarcoidosis have refractory illness that is associated with considerable morbidity and potential mortality. These patients often have CNS mass lesions, hydrocephalus, or diffuse encephalopathy or vasculopathy. Patients with recurrent aseptic meningitis, cranial polyneuropathies, myopathy, or neuropathy may have a protracted course, but they generally do not die of the illness.

Corticosteroids may lead to improvement in radiographic features and pulmonary function. Patients with refractory neurosarcoidosis often require long-term high-dose corticosteroid therapy to control their symptoms. Methotrexate, cyclosporine, azathioprine, hydroxychloroquine, and infliximab have been used successfully in conjunction with corticosteroids. The use of these agents should be restricted to patients who require long-term treatment or those with CNS, cardiac, or other progressive disease refractory to systemic corticosteroid therapy. Fatalities usually occur because of progressive respiratory, CNS, or cardiac involvement.

REFERENCE

Thomas KW, Hunninghake GW. Sarcoidosis. *JAMA* 2003;**289**:3300-3.

History

For several months, a 74-year-old man noted mild occasional occipital headaches. While he was playing tennis, violent rotatory vertigo developed and he fell. He recovered but continued to complain of vertigo if he changed direction suddenly while walking. He also had noted loss of appetite, reduced energy, and a 10-lb weight loss in recent months. The patient worked in a nuclear reactor facility. Ten years earlier, he had had an operation for prostate cancer.

Examination

Neurologic examination showed hypometric saccades and horizontal nystagmus on right gaze. Also, the right palate elevated a bit less than the left, and tests of coordination demonstrated minimal right arm and leg ataxia.

Investigations

Magnetic resonance imaging (MRI) demonstrated an irregular, inhomogeneous, ring-enhancing, partially cystic mass in the medial aspect of the right cerebellar hemisphere, with mild adjacent edema (Figure). Radiographically, the differential diagnosis included a solitary metastasis of an unknown primary source versus an infratentorial glioma. Through a right suboccipital craniotomy, the mass was totally resected. Intraoperatively, the mass appeared to arise from cranial nerve X (vagus nerve), but it also was closely associated with cranial nerve XII (hypoglossal nerve).

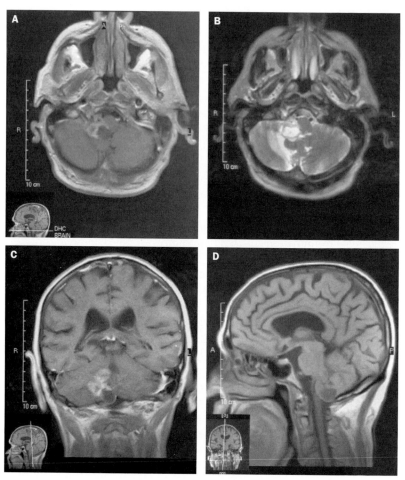

FIGURE. MRI demonstrates (*A* and *C*) a heterogenously enhancing mass in the right cerebellomedullary region, with the cystic component (hypointense area in *D*) exerting a mass effect on the medulla. *B*, Peritumoral edema, evident on this T$_2$-weighted image, contributes to the local mass effect.

Commentary by Dr. Joon H. Uhm

Histopathologic examination demonstrated that the tumor was a schwannoma. Although these tumors are associated more commonly with peripheral nerves, they account for approximately 8% of intracranial tumors. The cranial nerve classically associated with schwannomas is VIII (vestibulocochlear nerve), with bilateral involvement being pathognomonic for neurofibromatosis type 2 (NF2). In contrast, schwannomas affecting the lower cranial nerves (IX, X, XI) in the absence of NF2 are rare, constituting less than 3% of all intracranial schwannomas (less than 0.24% of all primary intracranial neoplasms). Moreover, even in rare instances in which lower cranial nerves are affected, most of the tumors involve the jugular foramen. In our patient, the tumor was located more proximally along cranial nerve X in the cerebellomedullary cistern. This is an extremely rare location for schwannomas, and fewer than 15 such cases in the absence of NF2 have been reported.

Because of the rarity of schwannomas in this location, more ominous neoplasms were considered preoperatively in our patient, especially in the context of his advanced age, constitutional symptoms, weight loss, and possible exposure to radiation (nuclear facility). With the mass effect on the medulla, the decision was to resect rather than to biopsy the mass to palliate his symptoms and to make a histologic diagnosis. Postoperatively, the patient had an excellent recovery, with marked improvement in his level of energy and resolution of the mild hemiataxia. With confirmation of the diagnosis of schwannoma, the patient's personal and family histories were reassessed for possible NF2, but no compelling evidence to support NF2 could be found. Follow-up MRI studies have not shown evidence of tumor recurrence.

With rare exceptions, schwannomas are slowly growing benign tumors, and surgery is curative in virtually every case. Histologically, the tumor consists of characteristic spindle-shaped neoplastic Schwann cells. In a given tumor, the structure can be heterogeneous, with areas of relatively compact cellularity and nuclear pallisading (Antoni A pattern) contrasting with areas of reduced cellularity consisting of loosely textured tumor cells (Antoni B pattern). The degree of cellularity does not appear to influence prognosis because tumors that have predominantly or exclusively the hypercellular and compact (Antoni A) pattern (termed "cellular schwannoma") have not been reported to have a clinically malignant course.

Although the degree of cellularity is not prognostic, the presence of pigmentation that characterizes melanotic schwannomas may portend a worse outcome, with approximately 10% of melanotic schwannomas undergoing malignant transformation. These patients require, at the very least, close postoperative imaging follow-up, and some of them receive postoperative adjuvant radiation treatment. Melanotic schwannomas also can be associated with the genetic syndrome Carney's complex, an autosomal dominant syndrome consisting of pigmented schwannoma associated with lentiginous facial pigmentation, myxoma, and endocrine hyperactivity (typically, Cushing's syndrome).

In addition to Carney's complex, schwannomas are better known for their association with NF2, which is diagnosed on the basis of bilateral cranial nerve VIII schwannomas or fulfillment of the diagnostic criteria. The gene for NF2, the tumor suppressor *merlin/schwannomin*, is located on the long arm of chromosome 22. Mutations of this gene have been observed in approximately 60% of schwannomas. When multiple schwannomas occur in the absence of other NF2-related features, the kindreds are labeled as "schwannomatosis," a newly described syndrome.

In summary, vagal schwannomas in the cerebellomedullary region are exceptionally rare and radiographically can mimic a higher grade tumor, such as a solitary metastasis or glioma. Surgical resection secured the diagnosis of schwannoma and improved the patient's neurologic status.

REFERENCE

Sharma RR, Pawar SJ, Dev E, *et al.* Vagal schwannoma of the cerebello-medullary cistern presenting with hoarseness and intractable tinnitus: a rare case of intra-operative bradycardia and cardiac asystole. *J Clin Neurosci* 2001;8:577-80.

History

Two weeks before evaluation, a 35-year-old man awoke with discomfort in his right shoulder. Within a few days, the pain worsened significantly and involved both shoulders. He noted winging of the right scapula. The pain was worse at night and was associated with a feeling of neck stiffness. Four days before evaluation, he noted a painful rash across his left shoulder. Because of superficial tenderness of the affected area, he avoided contact of the area by clothing. He had a past history of Crohn's disease.

Examination

The neurologic examination demonstrated only winging of the right scapula (Figure). There was a vesicular rash on an inflammatory red base overlying the left scapula.

Investigations

The results of nerve conduction studies were normal. There were spontaneous fibrillation potentials but no motor unit potentials under voluntary control in the right serratus anterior muscle. Cerebrospinal fluid analysis showed five nucleated cells per microliter (85% lymphocytes, 9% mononuclear cells, 3% neutrophils, and 3% macrophages), increased protein concentration (1.5 x normal value), and a normal glucose level. Culture of the vesicular lesion was negative for herpes simplex and varicella-zoster virus (VZV).

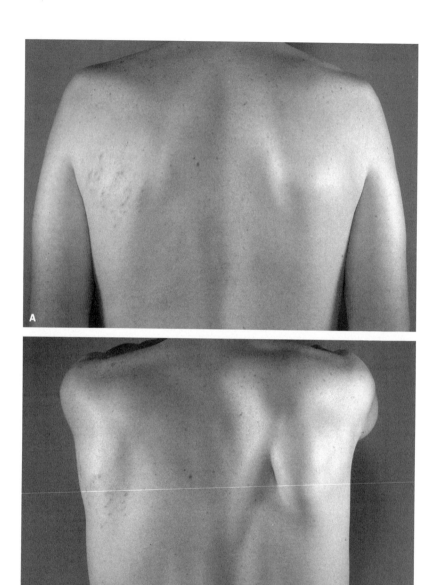

FIGURE. *A*, Zoster (shingles) rash affecting the left T4 dermatome. *B*, Weakness of the right serratus anterior muscle demonstrated by winging of the right scapula as the patient thrusts forward the outstretched upper limb against resistance (see color insert).

Commentary by Dr. Allen J. Aksamit

Segmental zoster paresis is a recognized complication of herpes zoster (shingles). This may occur in patients of any age, but the elderly and immunosuppressed are most vulnerable. The incidence of segmental weakness occurring in association with zoster infection has not been frequently studied. In a review of 1,210 cases of herpes zoster at Mayo Clinic, Thomas and Howard found 61 (5%) cases of segmental zoster paresis. Most often, the segmental weakness is manifest in the same myotome as the dermatome affected. Because a thoracic dermatome is usually affected, segmental weakness in the same myotome may not be manifested clinically. When herpes zoster affects cervical, lumbar, or trigeminal dermatomes, the clinical expression of segmental weakness may be demonstrated more easily. A better known example of segmental zoster paresis is Ramsay Hunt syndrome, with facial nerve paresis and zoster vesicles present on the ipsilateral ear pinna, the sensory representation of the facial nerve.

Herpes zoster is a reactivation infection by VZV in the dorsal root ganglion. This presents cutaneously after axonal transport of the virus in a "centrifugal" direction from infected dorsal root ganglion neurons to the skin. The dorsal root ganglion lies close to the ventral motor root in the intervertebral foramen. Presumably, segmental weakness is expressed in the same myotome as the affected dermatome by viral spread to and inflammation of the adjacent ventral root, although the precise mechanism of this has not been well studied. VZV may also spread in a "centripetal" direction from the reactivation site in the dorsal root ganglion, accounting for the occurrence of zoster myelitis or meningoencephalitis complicating shingles.

In our patient, the segmental weakness became manifest at a site remote from the sensory ganglion origin of the infection. The clinical expression of herpes zoster was the left T4 dermatome, whereas the segmental weakness was mononeuritis in the right long thoracic nerve. The presumed direction of spread is centripetal to cerebrospinal fluid pathways and then centrifugal along the perineurium or vasa nervosum. This infection affected the motor nerve remote from the site of the primary dorsal root ganglion reactivation. Because centripetal and centrifugal spread may occur at different rates, the remote motor paresis may precede the appearance of the rash, as in this case. In the review of Thomas and Howard, remote segmental zoster paresis occurred in 2 of 61 cases (3%) of segmental paresis. Theoretically, any motor nerve root or motor nerve may be vulnerable.

Culture of skin lesions is notoriously insensitive for demonstrating the growth of VZV. Polymerase chain reaction amplification of a specimen from pathologic skin vesicles or aspirate is the preferred and more sensitive method for confirming VZV.

Treatment, as for uncomplicated herpes zoster, should be antiviral therapy active against VZV. Oral acyclovir, 800 mg five times daily for 7 to 14 days, is required for suppression of VZV. There are no prospective studies of treatment of segmental paresis to establish whether intravenous acyclovir, with higher blood levels than oral acyclovir, is more effective at improving the prognosis of segmental weakness. Because of superior oral absorption, valacyclovir, 1,000 mg three times daily, or famciclovir, 500 mg three times daily for 7 to 14 days, is recommended. Whether prolonged therapy is more beneficial for recovery is uncertain, but some infectious disease specialists recommend a 21-day course. Prognosis has not been well studied, but according to earlier reviews, motor recovery is possible in 80% of patients. However, presumably because of inflammatory or infectious axonal injury, motor deficit may be long lasting. Immunosuppression may be associated with a worse prognosis. Our patient had not experienced improvement when he was examined 7 weeks after his initial presentation.

REFERENCE

Thomas JE, Howard FM Jr. Segmental zoster paresis—a disease profile. *Neurology* 1972;**22**:459-66.

History

A 58-year-old man had become aware of increasing forgetfulness over the previous 12 to 18 months. Both his wife and employer were aware of his increasing tendency to make more notes for himself and to rely more extensively on his secretary. He was a professional who regularly dealt with the public and now was having difficulty remembering the names of acquaintances and recent conversations. His wife also noted that if he was distracted, he might forget to bring groceries into the house after shopping. Otherwise, he functioned normally without any compromise in his activities of daily living. His family history was notable for his mother dying of cancer in her 80s several years after a dementing illness developed.

Examination

On mental status testing with the Kokmen Short Test of Mental Status, the patient scored 35 of 38 points, losing 2 points on delayed verbal recall and 1 point on complex attention. The rest of the neurologic examination was notable for a mild tremor and slightly brisk reflexes but not of pathologic significance.

Investigations

The results of routine laboratory tests, including a complete blood count, electrolytes, glucose, liver and kidney function, thyroid function, vitamin B_{12}, folate, and syphilis serologic testing, were unremarkable. Magnetic resonance imaging, with use of a temporal lobe volume protocol, showed mild atrophy of the hippocampal formation bilaterally. Fluorodeoxyglucose positron emission tomography showed a mild reduction in metabolism in the anterior and medial temporal lobes and in the mid-posterior parietal lobes bilaterally, which was somewhat worse on the left. Neuropsychologic testing documented an impairment in delayed verbal and nonverbal recall, with relative preservation of attention, executive function, language, processing speed, and visuospatial skills.

Commentary by Dr. Ronald C. Petersen

MCI is a transitional state between the cognitive changes of normal aging and very early dementia. As the field of aging and dementia moves toward early identification of cognitive symptoms, MCI has become an area of active research. Most clinicians believe that neurodegenerative processes evolve over years and perhaps decades. Thus, the concept of an intermediate stage of impairment between normal aging and early dementia needs to be clarified.

MCI has evolved to represent this transitional zone (Figure). According to recent research, MCI can be classified into three subtypes: 1) *amnestic MCI*, in which the person has a memory impairment out of proportion to performance in other cognitive areas; 2) *multidomain MCI*, in which the person has a slight impairment in several cognitive domains, for example, language, attention, executive function, and visuospatial skills with or without a memory impairment, although these deficits are mild and not sufficient to constitute dementia; and 3) *single non-memory domain MCI*, in which the person is impaired in a non-memory area in relative isolation to the other cognitive domains. All these forms of MCI presume that the person is neither normal nor demented and that functional activities are largely preserved. As the Figure shows, the various subtypes of MCI have different outcomes. As with any discussion of differential diagnoses in neurology, the eventual outcome depends on the clinical presentation and suspected cause of the clinical symptoms.

After the clinical subtype has been identified, the clinician can determine the putative cause of the symptoms. If the history is one of an insidious onset and gradual progression and other causes have been ruled out, the etiology is likely degenerative. Therefore, if the clinical subtype is amnestic MCI and it likely has a degenerative etiology, it most likely represents prodromal Alzheimer's disease. The other clinical subtypes may have various causes and may be precursors of other dementing conditions such as frontotemporal dementia or dementia with Lewy bodies. For example, if the MCI presentation is the single non-memory domain type with impairments in insight, social behavior, and executive function, this clinical subtype of MCI may progress to frontotemporal dementia. Alternatively, if an early presentation of this type of MCI includes extrapyramidal symptoms, visual hallucinations, a rapid eye movement behavior disorder of sleep, and impairments in processing speed and visuospatial skills, this phenotype may be the forme fruste of dementia with Lewy bodies.

Most research has been performed on the amnestic subtype of MCI because the rate at which these persons progress to Alzheimer's disease is 10% to 15% per year, which is in contrast to the incidence rate of 1% to 2% per year for the general population 65 years and older. Thus, MCI and its subtypes are important to identify because of the high likelihood of progression to a more severe degree of cognitive impairment. The transition from MCI to clinically probable Alzheimer's disease can be subtle. Generally, when the cognitive impairment spreads beyond memory to involve other cognitive domains, for example, executive function, in a clinically important fashion and functionally impairs the activities of daily living, the person is likely to have crossed the threshold for the clinical diagnosis of Alzheimer's disease. It must be emphasized that this is a clinical diagnosis: no rating scales or instruments with cutoff scores can make this determination for the clinician.

Although the neuropathologic features of amnestic MCI are not well known, studies have indicated that most of the patients have neuropathologic abnormalities of medial temporal lobe structures, which account for the memory impairment, in addition to various other contributing abnormalities. The most frequent type of medial temporal lobe lesion includes neurofibrillary tangles with various degrees of amyloid deposition. Generally, the amyloid deposition in the neocortex is the diffuse type rather than the neuritic form, which is characteristic of Alzheimer's disease. In most cases, there are not sufficient neuritic plaques in the neocortex to constitute the diagnosis of definite Alzheimer's disease. In addition to these findings, some cases have vascular changes, argyrophilic grains, and, uncommonly, hippocampal sclerosis. Most persons do not have the neuropathologic substrate of Alzheimer's disease at the time of MCI; instead, they have the appearance of being in transition to that condition.

Currently, no treatment is available for MCI, but several clinical trials are under way. These trials include evaluations of virtually all the acetylcholinesterase inhibitors approved by the U.S. Food and Drug Administration for the treatment of Alzheimer's disease, including donepezil, rivastigmine, and galantamine. Other trials are investigating antioxidants (vitamin E), anti-inflammatory agents (rofecoxib), glutamate receptor modulators (ampakines), and nootropics (piracetam). Also, agents that alter amyloid processing such as immunotherapy and β and γ secretase inhibitors are being considered. If any of these is successful, the results will underscore the importance of early recognition of intermediate forms of cognitive impairment such as MCI.

The patient described above met the criteria for amnestic MCI. He had a notable deficit in memory function, yet other cognitive skills and functional abilities were preserved. His neuropsychologic profile corroborated this clinical impression, and the results of imaging studies were suggestive of an early Alzheimer-like process. Management at this time would involve counseling for the implications of this condition for the future and a modification of lifestyle variables. As more information about the outcomes of clinical trials becomes available, he may be a candidate for early intervention.

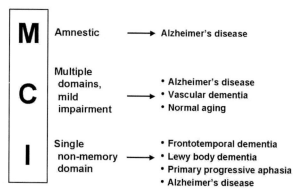

FIGURE. Clinical subtypes of mild cognitive impairment and their ultimate clinical outcome. (Modified from Petersen RC. In: Petersen RC, Ed. *Mild Cognitive Impairment: Aging to Alzheimer's Disease*. New York: Oxford University Press; 2003:1-14. By permission of Mayo Foundation for Medical Education and Research.)

REFERENCE

Petersen RC, Ed. *Mild Cognitive Impairment: Aging to Alzheimer's Disease*. New York: Oxford University Press; 2003.

Index

acanthocytes 157
acid α-glucosidase activity (GAA) 176
acid maltase 176
   deficiency 128
acquired immunodeficiency syndrome 151
acute disseminated encephalomyelitis (ADEM) 99
adenoid cystic carcinoma of the parotid gland 138
adult acid maltase deficiency 176
adult polyglucosan body disease (APBD) 47
adult-onset GM_2 gangliosidoses 7
AL amyloidosis 112
Alexander's disease
   adult 43
   infantile 43
αβ-crystallin 43
α-lipoprotein deficiency 103
alpha-synucleinopathies 83
Alzheimer's disease 206
   changes 84
amphiphysin-IgG 35
amyotrophic lateral sclerosis (ALS)-dementia complex 67
aneurysmal subarachnoid hemorrhage 91
Angelman's syndrome 58
angle-closure glaucoma
   acute 154
   intermittent 154
ANNA-1 (also known as "anti-Hu") 35
ANNA-3 36
anterior communicating artery aneurysm 91
anterior communicating artery aneurysm paraparesis syndrome 91
anterior opercular syndrome (Foix-Cavany-Marie syndrome) 63
anti-Ma 36
Ashkenazi Jewish population 158
asymmetric cortical degeneration 3
autism 58
autoimmune thyroiditis 71
autonomic neuropathy 35
autonomic polyneuropathy 112

fungal disease 195

motor neuron disease 8
Muckle-Wells syndrome 118
multifocal motor neuropathy 125
multiple sclerosis 121, 151
multiple system atrophy 83
mycobacterial infections 195
myeloneuropathy 133
myofibrillar myopathy 128
myokymia 24
myotonic discharges 176
myotonic dystrophy 128

neonatal-onset multisystem inflammatory disease (NOMID) 116, 118
neurofibromatosis type 2 (NF2) 199
neuromyelitis optica (Devic's disease) 75, 190
neuromyotonia 24
neuropathic pain 27
neurosarcoidosis 195
nonmetastatic lung carcinoma 86
norepinephrine 141, 143
normal aging 206
Notch3 gene 99

occipital condyle syndrome 11
oculomasticatory myorhythmia (OMM) 40
opercular syndrome 62
opsoclonus-myoclonus 35
optic disk swelling 147
optic neuropathy 172
oropharyngeal dysphagia 175
orthostatic hypotension 141
orthostatic tremor 51
osteosclerotic myeloma 147

P/Q voltage-gated calcium channel (VGCC) antibodies 184
paraneoplastic autonomic neuropathy 35, 112
paraneoplastic limbic encephalitis 35
paraneoplastic optic neuritis 189
paraneoplastic subacute encephalomyeloradiculoneuropathy 189
paraprotein-associated demyelinating neuropathies 125
Parkinson's disease 51, 83, 157, 158
paroxysmal spells 44

type II glycogenosis (glycogen storage disease [GSD-II]) 176
tyrosine hydroxylase 159

UBE3A 59
uveocyclitis 151

vagus nerve 86
  stimulation 15
varicella-zoster virus (VZV) 201
venous hypertension 108
verrucous angiomas 147
vesicular acetylcholine transporter 169
vesicular proton pump 169

weakness of the right serratus anterior muscle 202
Wegener's granulomatosis 195
Whipple's disease 39
white fingernails 147
Wilson's disease 133, 135

xanthelasmas 165

zinc 132, 133
zoster (shingles) 202
  meningoencephalitis 203
  myelitis 203
  segmental weakness 203